the total
suspended bodyweight
training workout

TRADE SECRETS OF A PERSONAL TRAINER

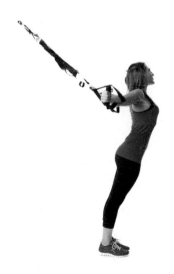

Note
Whilst every effort has been made to ensure that the content of this book is as technically accurate and as sound as possible, neither the author nor the publishers can accept responsibility for any injury or loss sustained as a result of the use of this material.

Published by Bloomsbury Publishing Plc
50 Bedford Square
London WC1B 3DP
www.bloomsbury.com

First edition 2013

ISBN (print): 978 1 4088 3258 5
ISBN (epub): 978 1 4081 9380 8
ISBN (epdf): 978 1 4081 9381 5

A CIP catalogue record for this book is available from the British Library.

Acknowledgements
Cover photograph © ESC Creative LLP www.esccreative.com
Inside photographs © ESC Creative LLP for all exercise photos
and © Shutterstock for filler photos
Commissioning Editor: Charlotte Croft
Editor: Sarah Cole
Cover and textual designer: James Watson
Illustrations by David Gardner and Mark Silver

This book is produced using paper that is made from wood grown in managed, sustainable forests. It is natural, renewable and recyclable. The logging and manufacturing processes conform to the environmental regulations of the country of origin.

Typeset in 10.25pt on 13.5pt URWGroteskLig by Margaret Brain, Wisbech

Printed and bound in India by Replika Press Pvt Ltd
10 9 8 7 6 5 4 3 2 1

the total
suspended bodyweight
training workout

TRADE SECRETS OF A PERSONAL TRAINER

STEVE BARRETT

BLOOMSBURY
LONDON • NEW DELHI • NEW YORK • SYDNEY

disclaimer and advisory

Before attempting any form of exercise, especially that which involves lifting weights, always ensure you have a safe working environment. Ensure that the floor surface you are on is non-slip and do not stand on any rugs or mats that could move when you exercise. Also, clear your exercise space of items that could cause you harm if you collided with them; this includes furniture, pets and children. Pay particular attention to the amount of clearance you have above your head and remember that for some of the exercise moves you will be raising your hands and the weights above head height, so keep away from doorways and light fittings.

The information, workouts, health related information and activities described in this publication are practised and developed by the author and should be used as an adjunct to your understanding of health and fitness and, in particular, strength training. While physical exercise is widely acknowledged as being beneficial to a participant's health and well-being, the activities and methods outlined in this book may not be appropriate for everyone. It is fitness industry procedure to recommend all individuals, especially those suffering from disease or illness, to consult their doctor for advice on their suitability to follow specific types of activity. This advice also applies to any person who has experienced soft tissue or skeletal injuries in the past, those who have recently received any type of medical treatment or are taking medication and women who are, or think they may be, pregnant.

The author has personally researched and tried all of the exercises, methods and advice given in this book on himself and with many training clients. However, this does not mean these activities are universally appropriate and neither he nor the publishers are, therefore, liable or responsible for any injury, distress or harm that you consider may have resulted from following the information contained in this publication.

contents

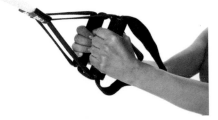

1 the basics of exercising with a suspension system

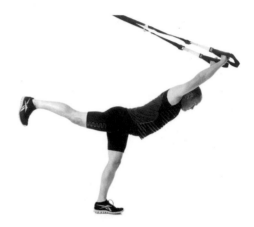

the S.A.F.E. trainer system
(Simple, Achievable, Functional Exercise)

. . . .

We need to exercise our bodies in a way that is achievable, effective and, most of all, sustainable so that the method becomes part of our lifestyle, rather than an inconvenience.

In a perfect world everyone would be able to lift their own bodyweight above their head, have ideal body-fat levels and be able to run a four-minute mile. Any one of these goals is achievable if you are highly motivated and have very few other commitments in your life, but the reality is that most people are so far off this state of perfection that the biggest challenge is either starting an exercise programme, or staying committed and engaged with a method of training for long enough to see any kind of improvement.

Exercise is in many ways a perfect product, because it has very few negative side effects, it is cheap to do and highly versatile. But so many high profile, quick-fix programmes and products make exercise sound easy, as though it is a magic wand that once waved will bring near instant results. And with the fitness industry constantly driven by innovation in products and methods, the diverse and sometimes bewildering amount of advice available makes it all too easy to be overwhelmed. The truth is that many training programmes and methods will theoretically work, but the level of commitment needed is so high that when you add in work and family responsibilities, stress and other demands upon time, most of us simply cannot stick to a plan.

I also find that those programmes which seem too good to be true usually have a series of components that are not explicit in the headline, but are required to achieve the spectacular results they boast about. So you sign up to a workout programme claiming: 'Instant fat loss – ultra 60 second workout!' only to find that to achieve the promised weight loss you have to go on an impossible 500-calories-a-day diet. These methods also assume that everybody is fairly perfect already; by this I mean they don't have any injuries, they are strong, mobile and flexible and have a cardiovascular system that will soak up anaerobic training from day one. If these people are out there, I don't see them walking up and down the average high street. There is a real need to approach fitness in a more down to earth, less sensationalist way. We need to exercise our bodies in a way that is achievable, effective and, most of all, sustainable so that the method becomes part of our lifestyle, rather than an inconvenience.

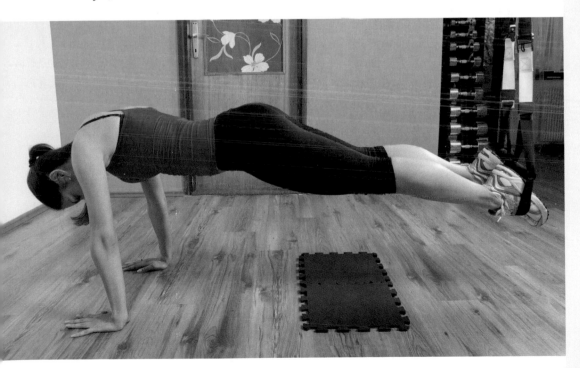

My S.A.F.E. trainer system (Simple, Achievable, Functional Exercise) is all of these things. It is based on 20 years of personal training experience, including many thousands of hours of coaching, lifting, running, jumping and stretching with people from all walks of life, from the average man or woman to elite athletes. My system respects the natural way that the body adapts to activity and creates a perfect physiological learning curve.

All S.A.F.E. trainer system moves develop stability, strength or power. If you're not familiar with these essential components of human performance, I am sure that you will recognise the saying: 'You have to walk before you can run'. This is the epitome of my approach, because when a client says they want to run or jump, the first thing I have to establish as a personal trainer is that they are at least already at the walking stage. I consider stability to be the walking phase of human movement, as it teaches you the correct muscle recruitment patterns; strength the running phase, as it trains the body to do these moves against a greater force (resistance); and power the jumping phase, since it teaches you to add speed and dynamics to the movement.

This book focuses on all the positive reasons for using a suspension system and aims to help you enhance the results you get from the time you spend doing strength and conditioning training. When you get to the portfolio of exercises (see page 47) demonstrating the actual exercises (or 'moves' as I like to call them) you will find that, rather than just giving a list of exercises with a suspension system, I have focused on the moves that really work. There are hundreds of moves that can be done with a set of straps, but many of them are very similar to each other, ineffective or potentially dangerous. This book is all about combining skills and methods to create safe and effective fitness ideas to help you get the most out of the time you spend exercising.

You'll find that the majority of the exercises progress through three stages; I don't like to refer to these as easy, medium and advanced because in reality some of the changes are very subtle while on others you would really notice if you were to try all three versions back to back. Instead, the following three levels closely mirror the systematic approach athletes use in the weight training room and on the training field:

1 each move can be progressed or regressed by changing body position;
2 resistance is applied to the move;
3 the speed at which the move is performed is increased;

– or in fact a combination of all three.

how to use this book

To help you make sense of each suspension exercise and how it relates to my S.A.F.E. training system, each move is classified by its respective outcome, whether that is an increase in stability, strength or power, rather than the more subjective easy, medium and hard.

Training with a suspension system is not only safe but it is also a very efficient use of your time. Suspension systems have in a very short time become an indispensable tool, not just for the world of health and fitness, but also for sportsmen and women. The possibilities are endless, and no matter whether your goals are strength, mobility, balance, co-ordination or simply a desire for cosmetically firmer, more toned muscles, a suspension system can play a significant part in helping you to achieve them.

When I started to think about writing this book, the first thing I had to come to terms with is that there is a wide range of information available that sets out to teach you how to use suspension system equipment. Likewise, in my everyday

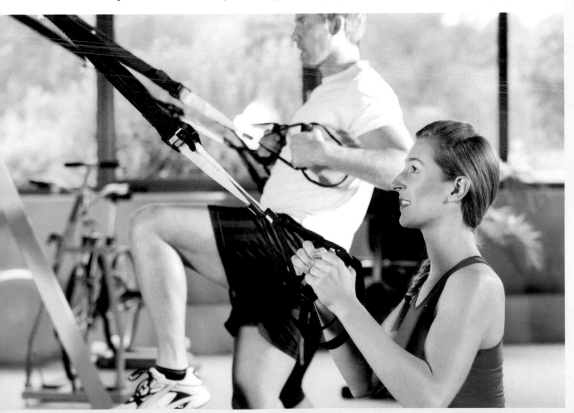

life as a personal trainer I know that my clients have access to information not only from myself, but from a wide range of sources such as the web, books and no doubt other personal trainers they come across in the gym, so I always aim to share my knowledge and experiences in a way that is useable, interesting and progressive. Interestingly, in the case of working out with suspension systems, I feel that much of the self-published information posted online is counter-productive because rather than being a learning resource much of the information comes in a 'one size fits all' format with the presenter's logic being 'if I can, you can' which frankly is never a good way to develop a training strategy.

As I have worked with many of my clients now for over a decade, clearly they find my approach productive and a worthwhile investment. With this in mind, my aim is to condense 25 years' experience of training my own body and, more importantly, 20 years' experience as a personal trainer and many thousands of hours of training the bodies of other people into this book.

Don't worry: this isn't an autobiography in which I wax lyrical about the celebrities and Premier League footballers I've trained. Yes, I have trained those types of people, but to me every client has the same goal for every training session: they want to get maximum results from the time they are prepared to invest in exercise. Every exercise I select for their session, therefore, has to have earned its place in the programme and every teaching point that I provide needs to be worthwhile and have a positive outcome. In essence, my teaching style could almost be described as minimalist. Now that the fitness industry enters its fourth decade, many of you will have accumulated a level of knowledge and information equal to some fitness professionals in the industry, so I don't go in for trying to show you how clever I am when all that is required are clear and concise instructions.

I learned this lesson many years ago when I was hired as personal trainer to a professor of medicine. There was absolutely nothing I could say about the function of the body that she didn't already know, but what I could do was assess her current level of ability and take her on the shortest, safest and most effective route to an improved level of fitness. Seventeen years on I am still finding new ways to help her enjoy and benefit from the time we spend training together.

The thought process and methods I use are based on my belief that everybody feels better when they build activity into their lives, but not everybody has the motivation and time to create the type of bodies we see on the covers of fitness magazines. When training my clients, I am ultimately judged on the results I deliver. These results can present themselves in many ways, for example, in the mirror or on the weighing scales, but I also aim to help my clients make sense of what we are doing together. I find when talking about any activity it is best to focus on the outcomes rather than use subjective classifications, such as beginner/ advanced, easy/hard. Therefore, to help you make sense of each activity you'll be doing with the suspension system, and how it relates to my S.A.F.E. training system, each move is classified by its respective outcome, whether that be an increase in stability, strength or power, rather than the more subjective easy, medium and hard.

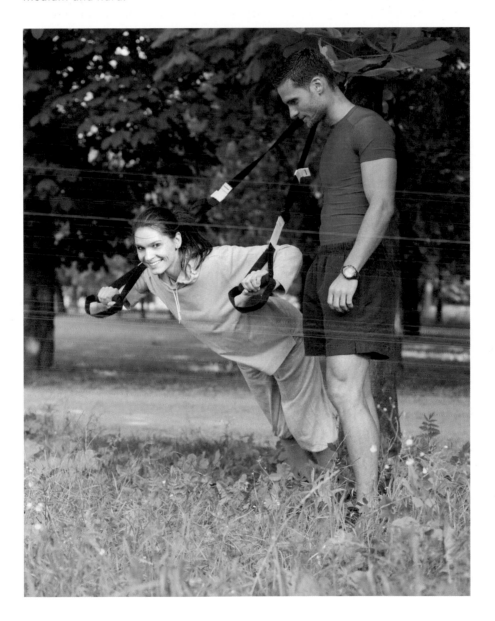

suspension system equipment overview

Gymnastic rings (plastic or wooden), ropes, one strap, two straps, lockable or 'saw-able' 'rip systems', pulleys ... the list of different types of equipment which can be used to suspend yourself from for the purpose of engaging and challenging the physical processes of the human body goes on and on.

All of these different suspension systems have individual characteristics which make them perform differently – some are very simple and others in my opinion are complicated and over-engineered. And for every piece of equipment there seems to be a 'fan club' that swears that their version is the best version, either because of its features, cost or sometimes just because they say so! My position on this is when I'm choosing equipment I want it to be the best available for the professional market, well-designed, robust and above all safe and effective.

In a very short period of time, using a suspension system to improve strength and athletic performance has become one of the most popular forms of exercise in gyms, sports clubs and at home. One product has been predominately responsible for this: the distinctive black and yellow TRX® Suspension Training system which without doubt is the most recognisable and widely used suspension system in the world (based on what I have seen on my extensive travels to fitness events globally). TRX®, under the direction of its founder Randy Hetrick, has not only created in my opinion the best suspension system available, but they have also delivered numerous instructor training workshops at the biggest fitness events in the world in an attempt to champion the safe and effective use of suspension techniques.

Thinking back, my very first experience of suspending my body and pulling my bodyweight up as a challenge would have been in PE lessons at school where our 'old school'-style gymnasium had ropes, rings and ladders that were suspended from the ceiling 25 feet above. At that age I was unstoppable and felt indestructible and 30 years on I can still remember climbing and hanging at the top of the ropes, so maybe – if you think laterally – suspension system training isn't necessarily new but rather it's certainly become more sophisticated. Fast forward to 2007 in San Francisco at the IHRSA (the International Health Racquet and Sportsclub Association) conference when I was making my way into the convention centre; there I notice a man with a set of black and yellow straps wrapped around a lamppost, where he was 'hanging' on the straps doing press-ups and rows. It was then and there that I had one of those 'Why didn't I think of that?' moments. That week, instead of returning from the USA with gadgets that I never use, I bought two TRX® suspension trainers which I brought back to the UK where they have been in constant use ever since.

key features of a suspension system

height adjustment

Whether you hang your suspension system from a frame, tree, door or any other solid, strong and secure object, you need to be able to adjust its length. If your suspension system has webbing and a carabiner, it is preferable to wrap the webbing around the fixing point rather than the carabiner itself; this helps minimise any movement of the strap at the anchor point.

adjustable straps

Having either buckles or sliders allows you to make quick and accurate adjustments to the length of the straps. Most of my chosen exercises require the straps

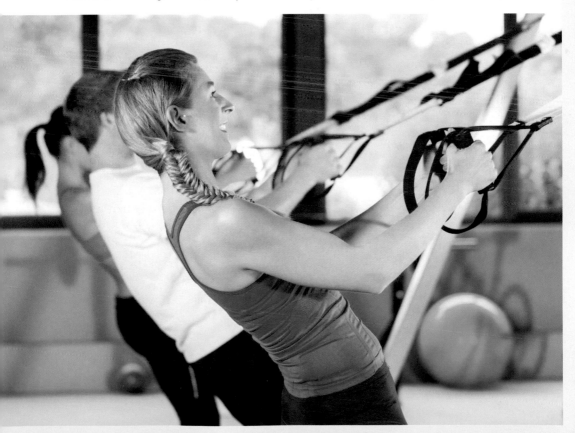

to be set at one of three lengths; these measurements are defined by how far from the floor the handles are: long = 6'' (15cm), medium = 12'' (30cm), and short = 18'' (45cm).

foot loops

There are products that combine the handles and foot loops into one component but personally I prefer them to be separate. You can support your feet either by your heels when lying on your back or by the bridge of your feet when lying on your front.

'locking' method

This feature enables you to use just one handle or foot strap when the other one has no load on it (this is only relevant if you have a single strap system). It also stops you from being able to do a 'sawing' action with the straps which is when pulling one end of the straps longer makes the other end become shorter (I know some trainers think this is a great exercise, but having tried the movement personally, I feel that while you do get some core activation, the sawing action from left to right just cancels out any productive upper body activity.) Different manufacturers have different components to achieve this, including the use of additional carabiners or pin locking systems, etc. My original 2007 TRX® suspension system didn't have the Locking Loop that they now feature in the updated version, so for single arm/leg exercises you needed to 'lace' the handles together to stop the single strap slipping through the attachment point.

 With so many different products on the market I have selected the exercises very carefully to ensure that, irrespective of which brand of suspension system you have, they will be applicable. As long as your equipment is adjustable, has two separate handles and foot loops then you can do all the moves in the portfolio.

every body is different

Just to be clear, any attempt to classify physical activity has to respect the fact that each human body responds to physical demands differently – there isn't an exact point where one move stops being beneficial for stability and switches over to being purely for strength. The transition is far more subtle and means that no matter which version of a move you are doing, you will never be wasting your time.

truly personalised intensity

With other types of fitness equipment it is easy to quantify and adjust the 'intensity' level – with cardio equipment such as bikes and treadmills you can go faster or add an incline to the challenge, with free weights you simply select a heavier weight to increase the difficulty. With suspension systems, adjusting the length of the straps is only the start of the personalisation process because variables will manipulate the intensity of every repetition. These include: user height, length of limbs, bodyweight, touch-points, Suspension Spiral position, the Vertical/Floor angle (V/F angle), stance, and of course the strap length.

user height

Obviously your height is a fixed entity and can't be changed; however, if you are working out with other people, it's common to compare your ability to theirs so bear in mind that because of the effects of physics some exercises will seem easier to shorter individuals (e.g. press-ups) because of their weight-to-height ratio and the length of their limbs.

length of limbs

Again this is a fixed entity (and if you work out on your own, then you will never notice this), but if you take two people of very different heights and they stand the same distance from the anchor, their perception of how 'hard' the exercise is will differ. However, don't see this as being either a positive or a negative – simply apply all the information outlined in this personalisation section and you will get the best out of every exercise.

bodyweight

Your power-to-weight ratio is relevant but as our goal is exercise and not competition it isn't going to affect how you set up your suspension system (strap length and touch-points are far more relevant).

touch-points

This refers to any parts of your body that are in contact with a supporting surface (floor, handles or foot loops). The fewer touch-points you use the harder

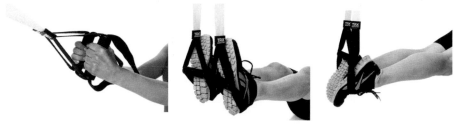

the exercise becomes. For example, if you do a suspended row standing on two feet and row with both arms, it will be an easier exercise than doing a suspended row holding just one handle and standing on one foot. There is an intermediate stage as well going from four to three to two touch-points when you use a split stance (see page 17).

suspension spiral position (SS)

SS is a reference system that lets users of suspension systems plot the appropriate position on the floor for their touch-points. Imagine a spiral radiating out from below the anchor point. Each loop of the spiral represents a regression of intensity for exercises like rows and presses. For example, when performing a row, having your feet directly below the anchor point will present the most challenging version of this move; standing the maximum distance (length of straps) from the anchor will create the easiest version.

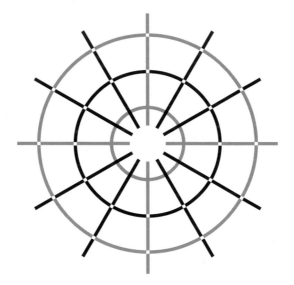

vertical/floor (V/F) angle

In addition to the Suspension Spiral position, the angle of your body in relation to the vertically hanging straps and the floor has a reference system to describe the angle of the user's body. Standing up straight is equal to a 90 degree V/F; as you lean towards the floor, your body and the floor create more acute angles. You will find that the exercise intensity increases significantly when you perform exercises at the smaller, more acute angles (e.g. 30 degree V/F). In the description of the moves, I refer to most of the angles as being 70, 45 and 30 degrees. Just remember, these are guidelines and for true personalisation you can adjust them to suit your ability and objectives.

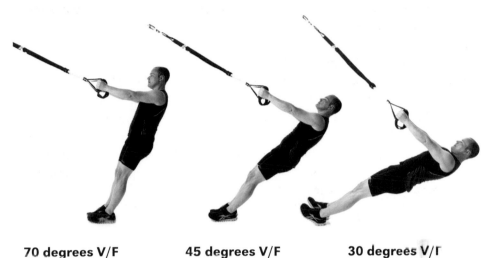

70 degrees V/F   **45 degrees V/F**   **30 degrees V/F**

stance

For many years I have been teaching 'core activation' to personal trainers using what I call the 'don't let me move you' method; this method also demonstrates perfectly how touch-points relate to exercise intensity with a suspension system. Most of the standing suspension system moves can be progressed and regressed by changing the foot position from two feet wide to two feet split to a single foot balance. It works best if you have a person to actually push against you, but if you are on your own you can still get a feel for the drill by standing in the pictured positions and twisting side to side:

In a 'wide and parallel stance', you will feel most stable and therefore place the fewest demands on your core stabilisers and other skeletal muscles.

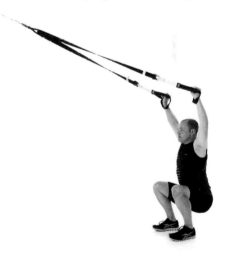

wide stance

In a 'split stance', you will feel less balanced and stable and therefore automatically engage your core stabilisers and other skeletal muscles more.

In a 'one foot balance', your balance will be at its most challenged and therefore you will encourage maximum activity from your core stabilisers and other skeletal muscles.

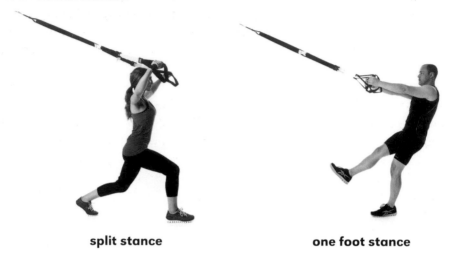

split stance   **one foot stance**

strap length

Changing the strap length can make the same exercise feel very different and all the moves have the suggested strap length listed next to the moves. As a means of changing the intensity of an exercise, it's quicker to change your foot position and/or the V/F angle.

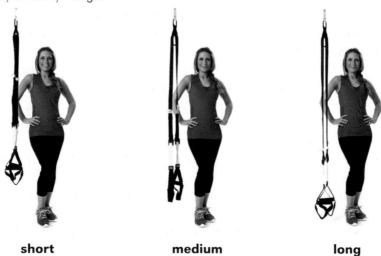

short   **medium**   **long**

don't skip the moves

Human nature might lead you to think that the way to achieve the quickest results would be to skip the 'easy' stability and strength moves and start on day one with the power versions. Overcoming this instinct is fundamental for banishing the 'old school approach' of beating up the body every training session, rather than using your training time wisely. My approach is about quality and not quantity. For a personal trainer to take this approach it requires true confidence and belief in the system, as some clients (particularly men) feel that they should be 'working hard' every session. This, I feel, is a situation unique to fitness training. In no other sport or activity would you set out to teach the body to cope with a new skill or level of intensity by starting with the high intensity or fastest version. For example, if you are learning to play golf, you don't start by trying to hit the ball a long way – rather you start by simply trying to make contact and hit it in the right direction. Or how about tennis? When learning to serve, if all you do is hit the ball as hard as you can, it is unlikely that any shot will ever stay within the lines of the court and therefore count. In all cases quality and the development of skill is the key to success.

mixing it up

The phenomenal success, availability and versatility of suspension systems have triggered a need to think about human movement in a completely new way. Today personal trainers, coaches and instructors think very differently about exercise compared to just ten years ago – this new mindset and way of thinking is responsible for the proliferation of the word 'functional' being used to describe exercise that has a direct relationship with the way we move in everyday life or during sporting activities. In just one decade the trend has gone from doing much of our strength training on machines that moved in straight lines to trying to incorporate the body's three planes of motion (sagittal, frontal and transverse) into all our conditioning exercises by using both improved weight machines and of course the huge selection of functional training products now available: sagittal involves movements from left to right of the body's centre line; frontal (coronal) involves movements which are forward and backward from the centre line; and transverse which are movements that involve rotation. The reality is these planes of motion never occur independently of each other so the best way to ensure you are working through all three planes is to create exercises that incorporate bending and twisting rather than to look at joint movements in isolation.

Before the fitness industry started to think with a 'functional' mindset it wasn't unusual to discourage any type of twisting during a workout; the introduction of functional training equipment and in particular suspension systems has evoked a completely different approach where we now actively look for ways to incorporate all the planes of motion into everything we do. The multi-plane moves don't altogether replace isolation moves that still have an important role to play (particularly if you are trying to overload and bulk up individual muscles). These isolation moves are generally good for overloading and challenging an individual muscle to adapt and react to the challenges of exercise, but working muscles one at a time leaves you with a body full of great individual muscle, when what you actually need are muscles that work as a team and in conjunction with other muscles that surround them. For example, despite most of the classic free weight exercises being integrated movements (i.e. they work more than one set of muscles at a time), the vast majority of free weight moves involve no rotation of the spine (through the transverse plane) and therefore don't train the body for the reality of everyday, where we constantly rotate at the same time as bending, pushing or pulling against external forces. Working muscles one at a time is not what a suspension system session sets out to do – our approach is ultimately 'all the muscles all of the time'. Even when the moves are highly targeted at smaller muscle groups such as the pecs and the triceps, being suspended enables them to be 'functional' rather than isolated, because in addition to the muscles being intentionally targeted, the moves have the additional benefit of directing force through the spine and lumbopelvic region and therefore activating the core stabilisers in a way that wouldn't occur if the same muscles were worked by using free weight or machines, either seated or standing.

Until the late 1990s not a second thought was given to the muscles that we now refer to as 'core stabilisers'. When new products hit the market it is not unusual for them, for a short time at least, to be included in everything that personal trainers and instructors do. This was the case with 'core training' and for some time it was all-encompassing and there was a trend to do everything we had previously done on a bench or on the floor on the stability ball instead, or to adopt a super slow Mat pilates-style approach to movements. Thankfully the trend for suspension exercise came along long enough after that era for us to have realised that 'exercising' the core needs to be something that we integrate into our workouts, rather than making it the sole purpose of every exercise session. Working out with a suspension system has the fantastic appeal of being able to challenge muscle, energy systems, the circularity system and the nervous system (which stimulates core muscle activity) making it pretty unique and without peer in terms of a fitness solution – it manages to complement everything and at the same time compete with nothing.

the workouts

In the final section of the book you will find a series of workouts. They are designed to be realistic sessions that you can do on any day of the week, without the need for 'rest' days or anything more than a reasonable amount of space.

All the workouts are sequential, so in theory you could start with 15 minutes of stability moves and do every workout until you reach 30 minutes of power moves. This is, of course, the theory; in reality you will naturally find the right start point depending on how you do with the assessment (see 'Assess, don't guess' on page 28) and how much time you have available on a given day. Continue using that particular workout until you feel ready to move on. I would advise everybody to start with the stability sessions, then move onto strength and then finally power, but I also accept that some people will find that the stability and strength moves don't challenge them enough so they will dive into the power phase. Please bear in mind that, if this is how you plan on approaching the exercises in this book, you might be missing out on a valuable learning curve that the body would benefit from.

a resource for life

My aim is for this book to be an ongoing reference point, and I suggest reading the entire contents and then dipping into the specific areas that interest you, such as the training programmes or fitness glossary. I guarantee you'll discover nuggets of information that perhaps you knew a little about, but had never fully understood because they had been explained in such a way that left you confused. If fitness training is an important part of your life, or even your career, then I know this book will be a long-term resource and will help you get the most from the time you spend using your suspension system.

FAQs

When learning to train with a suspension system, there are a handful of important questions that I get asked all the time.

What are the main differences between different types of suspension systems?

As with all products, there are good and bad points. There has been a flood of products onto the market all claiming to be the best or unique in some way. The key features that stand out are that the suspension systems are made from either one single strap or two separate ones, and that on the single strap versions you can or can't perform a 'sawing' action – sawing means that the single strap moves freely through its anchoring point rather than being fixed. Personally, my preferred suspension system is the TRX®. The design is very logical; it only has features that add to the functionality of the product and its quality inspires confidence – which is important when you consider you will be relying on it to support your weight while you exercise (for more details on the specific components see the equipment overview on page 12.)

I tried suspension exercises at the gym but found them too hard. Are they only for super fit people?

No, this type of training is very inclusive. If you found the exercises too hard, I expect you were trying it out on your own. Check out the section where I talk about 'exercise intensity' and how to adjust it, and you should find that it's as simple as getting the straps the right length or putting your hands or feet in the correct position.

Are suspension exercises harder if you are heavy?

The beauty of this type of exercise is that almost every movement can be adapted, progressed and regressed to suit the individual's ability. But the straight answer to the question is 'yes'. If you are heavy because you are carrying a lot of fat, then some of the exercises will be harder. It should also be noted that the user's height will affect their perception of what is easy or hard because of the mechanical effects that occur when you have short or long levers (arms, legs, torso).

Can I make my own suspension equipment?

Yes, but I would rather you didn't. The internet is full of advice on how you can save money by going to the hardware store and buying nylon straps, ropes and pulleys, but in my opinion if you are going to hang your entire bodyweight from an item, I would prefer to know that the product has been designed and tested by people who make these things for a living and have to put a guarantee on them.

What is the best way to hang my suspension system?

Depending upon which type of suspension system you have, you will have a variety of options. Most gyms have suspension systems in them now and they should be hanging them from suitable anchoring points like an A-frame or wall-mounted fixture. It is unwise to hang a suspension system from a machine in the gym that has a weight stack, such as a lat pulldown machine, because while these machines are heavy, all of their weight is in the base and, therefore, if you pull it with a strap from an angle, it may become unstable.

At home, a door anchor can prove to be a good solution as can structural features such as beams and pillars – but, of course, before you start hanging off them, ensure that they are capable of taking the weight.

Outdoors, you are spoilt for choice as suspension systems can be hung from suitable trees, lamp posts and solid items in parks such as children's swings and climbing frames.

Will suspension exercise give me big muscles?

No, especially not if you are a woman. This is a question personal trainers are often asked about all types of strength training. The reality is that building muscle doesn't happen by accident and requires close attention to diet and exercise – not to mention that 99.9% of women don't produce enough testosterone naturally to grow extra muscle bulk. What suspension exercise can and will do is improve the tone, firmness, definition and mechanical strength of all the muscles that you use when exercising this way.

Does suspension exercise create better results than lifting weights and, if so, why?

Using machines, suspension systems or free weights for strength training will all have pros and cons. Machines do have the disadvantage that because you are often sitting on them you do not benefit from being able to activate 'core stabilisers', but they have the advantage of being able to overload muscles individually which can be the fastest way to increase strength. Free weights, especially dumbbells and kettlebells, can deliver fantastic functional strength gains, but I think that if, like many people, you are short of time, suspension fitness offers the most efficient use of time as it is very easy to exercise every muscle in the body quickly and effectively.

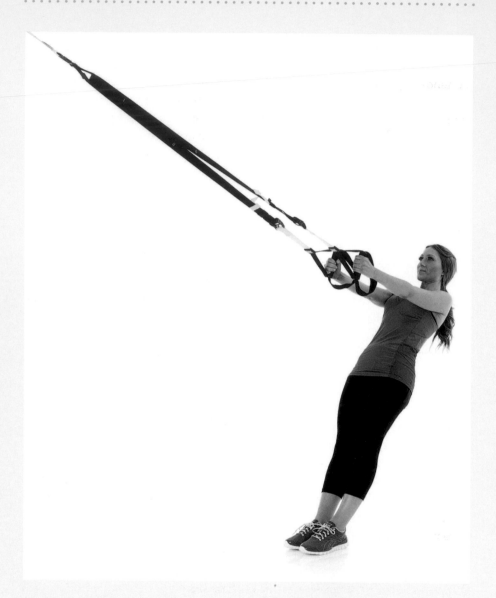

Does suspension exercise work the 'core'?

This subject can get very confusing so I thought it might help if I gave you my one-line description of what I think core training is.

Core training is: 'Exercise that develops strength and endurance for all muscles that protect the spine from damage and that function to produce dynamic movements'.

Or, the even shorter version: 'Exercise that makes you better at dealing with forces applied to the lumbopelvic region'.

As core training has evolved from physical therapy, where the main aim is to fix problems rather than achieve traditional fitness or cosmetic outcomes, there is a tendency to medicalise the use of suspension systems, gym balls and many other items of equipment that induce balance and muscle activation. However, since my aim is to increase fitness rather than to use your suspension system for therapy, I approach core training with the same attitude as I do all of my training: you need to walk before you can run. Therefore, if I find that a person is having issues with their balance, stability and overall quality of movement, I start right from the beginning, using the suspension system to re-train them to use (help activate) muscles and maintain postures at the lowest of intensity before moving on to what they would consider to be a 'workout'. But unlike many personal trainers who seem to revel in finding things wrong with their clients, I do not believe that everybody is bound to be in some way broken if they have not previously done 'core training'. Therefore, if you are healthy and injury free working the core does not need to feel like a visit to the doctor; it can and should be challenging and progressive but, above all, simple.

So, what are the core muscles and are they different from 'regular muscles'?

The lumbopelvic region consists of the deep torso muscles, transversus abdominis, multifidus, internal obliques and the layers of muscle and fascia that make up the pelvic floor. These are key to the active support of the lumbar spine, but unfortunately they are also the most vulnerable to injury if neglected. Using any kind of functional training equipment or methods to encourage the recruitment of these muscles is productive because the muscle activity is involuntary so, rather than having to tell the body to do something, it simply gets on with the work that is required. In fact, these muscles are recruited a split second before any movements of the limbs, which suggests that they actually anticipate the force that will soon be going through the lumbar spine.

Can I do suspension exercise outdoors?

Yes, but make sure that whatever you hang your suspension system from is strong enough to take your weight and also ensure that the floor space around you doesn't have anything that may cause you injury.

find your starting point

Before starting any exercise programme, test your body against the fitness checklist: mobility, flexibility, muscle recruitment and strength.

Before you think about grabbing a suspension system you need to establish what your starting point is, i.e. your current level of fitness, mobility, flexibility and strength. Every first consultation with a new personal training client revolves around the wish list of goals they hope to achieve. This list inevitably combines realistic goals with entirely unrealistic aims. Invariably people focus on their 'wants' rather than their 'needs' when goal-setting, and there is a big difference between the two mindsets. While 'wanting' could be considered a positive attitude, it will never overcome the need to slowly expose the body to processes that will change its characteristics and ability. Men in particular want to dive in at the most advanced stage of training, but it makes no sense to overload a muscle if your quality of movement is lacking.

realistic goal-setting

The secret of realistic goal-setting is understanding the difference between these two words:

Want (v) 'A desired outcome'
Need (n) 'Circumstances requiring some course of action'

By identifying your needs, your goals may not sound so spectacular but you are more likely to achieve better and longer term results, and your progress through the fitness process will be considerably more productive. Therefore, rather than thinking about the ultimate outcome, think instead of resolutions to the 'issues'.

fitness checklist

The checklist you need to put your body through before you start hanging on a set of suspension straps is very simple and logical. Our ability to lift or move weight (by which I mean bodyweight as well as external loads) relies on a combination of

- Mobility
- Flexibility

- Muscle recruitment
- Strength

If any of these vital components are neglected, it will have a knock-on effect on your progress. For example, while you may have the raw strength in your quadriceps to squat with a heavy weight, if you do not have a full range of motion in the ankle joints and sufficient flexibility in the calf muscles, then your squat will inevitably be of poor quality. Likewise, in gyms it is common to see men who have overtrained their chest muscles to such an extent that they can no longer achieve scapular retraction (they are round shouldered and therefore demonstrate poor technique in moves that require them to raise their arms above their heads).

This type of checklist is traditionally the most overlooked component of strength training and, while testing weight, body-fat levels and cardiac performance is now a regular occurrence in the fitness industry, the introduction of screening for quality of movement has taken a much longer time to become a priority, despite a self-administered assessment being as simple as looking in the mirror.

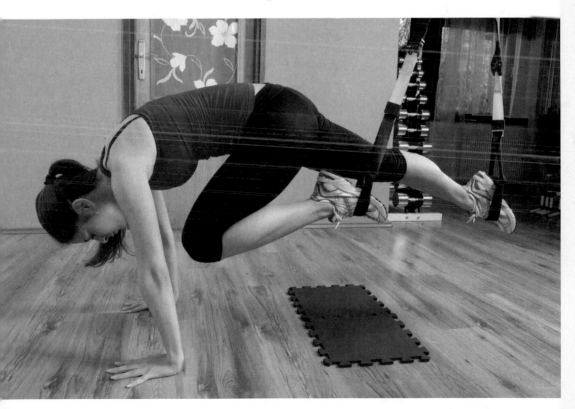

assess, don't guess

There is no better summary of the importance of our ability to move freely than in one of my favourite sayings: 'Use it or lose it'. This says it all – if you don't use the body to perform physical tasks, it will more likely deteriorate than just stay the same.

It may be no coincidence that assessing movement quality has grown in importance for athletes and fitness enthusiasts at the same pace as the popularity of functional training – rightly so, because if you don't assess yourself, then how can you know what areas of functionality you need to work on most? Before functional training became a key component of progressive fitness programmes, all progression was related to increasing duration, intensity and resistance, whereas now the quality of movement has become of equal importance.

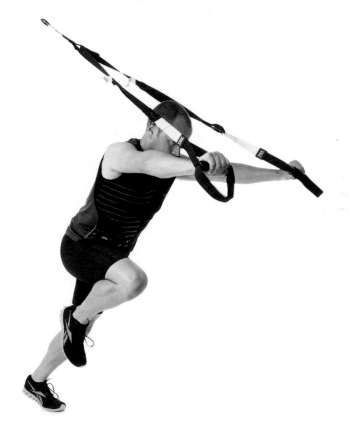

Today, the assessment of 'functional movement', or biomechanical screening, is its own specialised industry within the world of fitness. Those working in orthopaedics and conventional medical rehabilitation have always followed some form of standardised assessment where they test the function of the nerves, muscles and bones before forming an opinion of a patient's condition. Becoming a trained practitioner takes many years of study and practice. Not only must a practitioner gain knowledge of a wide spectrum of potential conditions, but just as importantly they must understand when and how to treat their patient, or when they need to refer them to other colleagues in the medical profession. Having been subjected to and taught many different approaches to movement screening, in my mind, the challenge isn't establishing there is something 'wrong', but knowing what to do to rectify the issue.

mobility and flexibility

The most common problem limiting quality of movement in the average person is a lack of mobility and flexibility, which can be provisionally tested using the standing twist and the overhead squat assessment (see pages 30–34).

To understand why mobility is key to human movement, think how, as babies, we start to move independently. We are born with mobility and flexibility, then we progressively develop stability, balance and then increasing levels of strength. As we get older we may experience injuries, periods of inactivity and, to some extent, stress, which all contribute towards a progressive reduction of mobility. There is no better summary of the importance of mobility than in one of my favourite sayings: 'Use it or lose it'. If you sit for extended periods or fail to move through the three planes of motion (see page 19), then you invariably become restricted in your motion. With this in mind, I hope you can see that lifting weights without first addressing mobility issues is like trying to build the walls of a house before you have completed the foundations.

The following two mobility tests challenge the entire length of the kinetic chain (actions and reactions to force that occur in the bones, muscles and nerves whenever dynamic motion or force is required from the body) and help to reveal if you are ready to move beyond bodyweight moves to begin adding the additional loads such as dumbbells. This test focuses on the key areas of the shoulders, the mid-thoracic spine, the pelvis, the knees, ankles and feet. Any limitation of mobility, flexibility or strength in these areas will show up as either an inability to move smoothly through the exercise or an inability to hold the body in the desired position.

Test 1 Standing twist

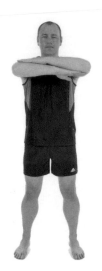 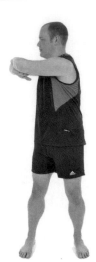

This is the less dramatic of the two mobility tests and serves to highlight if you have any pain that only presents when you move through the outer regions of your range of movement, and also if you have a similar range of motion between rotations on the left and right sides of your body.

- Stand with your feet beneath your hips.
- Raise your arms to chest height then rotate as far as you can to the right, noting how far you can twist.
- Repeat the movement to the left.
- Perform the movement slowly so that no 'extra twist' is achieved using speed and momentum.

You are trying to identify any pain and/or restriction of movement. If you find either, it might be the case that this reduces after a warm-up or a few additional repetitions of this particular movement. If you continue to experience pain, you should consider having it assessed by a physiotherapist or sports therapist.

Test 2 Overhead squat (OHS)

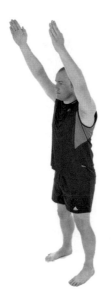 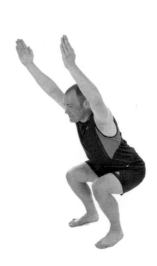

I've used the OHS test over 5000 times as part of my S.A.F.E. approach to exercise and I have found it to be the quickest and easiest way of looking at basic joint and muscle function without getting drawn into speculative diagnosis of what is and isn't working properly. If you can perform this move without any pain or restriction, you will find most of the moves in this book achievable. There is no pass or fail; rather you will fall into one of two categories: 'good' or 'could do better'. If you cannot achieve any of the key requirements of the OHS move, then it is your body's way of flagging up that you are tight and/or weak in that particular area. This, in turn, could mean you have an imbalance, pain or an untreated injury, which may not prevent you from exercising, but which you should probably get checked out by a physiotherapist or sports therapist.

Perform this exercise barefoot and in front of a full-length mirror so that you can gain maximum information from the observation of your whole body. Also refer to Table 1 for a list of key body regions to observe during this test. (This move also doubles up as a brilliant warm-up for many types of exercise including lifting weights.)

- Stand with feet pointing straight ahead and at hip width.
- Have your hands in the 'thumbs-up position' and raise your arms above your head, keeping them straight, into the top of a 'Y' position (with your body being

the bottom of the 'Y'). Your arms are in the correct position when they are back far enough to disappear from your peripheral vision.

- The squat down is slow and deep, so take a slow count of six to get down by bending your knees.
- The reason we go slowly is so you do not allow gravity to take over and merely slump down. Also, by going slowly you get a chance to see and feel how everything is moving through the six key areas.

The magic of this move is that you will be able to see and feel where your problem spots are and, even better, the test becomes the solution, because simply performing it regularly helps with your quality of movement. Stretch out any area that feels tight and aim to work any area that feels weak.

Table 1 Key body regions to observe in the overhead squat

Body region	Good position	Bad position
Neck		
Shoulders		
Mid-thoracic spine		

Body region	Good position	Bad position
Hips		
Knees		
Ankles and feet		

As you perform the OHS you are looking for control and symmetry throughout and certain key indicators that all is well.

- **Neck**: You keep good control over your head movements and are able to maintain the arm lift without pain in the neck.
- **Shoulders**: In the start position and throughout the move you are aiming to have both arms lifted above the head and retracted enough so that they are outside your peripheral vision (especially when you are in the deep part of the squat). In addition to observing the shoulders, look up at your arms to the hands – throughout the OHS you should aim to have your thumbs pointing behind you.
- **Mid-thoracic spine**: There is no instruction to keep your back straight, so in this area of the body you are looking for 'flow' rather than clunking movements.
- **Hips**: Imagine a straight line drawn directly down the centre of your body. Around the hips you are looking to see if you shift your weight habitually to one side, rather than keeping it evenly spread between both sides.

- **Knees**: The most common observation is the knees touching during the OHS, suggesting a weakness in the glutes. Less common is the knees parting, showing weakness in the inner thigh. Good technique is when your knees move forwards as you bend the legs. Note that clicking and crunching noises don't always suggest a problem unless they are accompanied by pain.
- **Ankles and feet**: The most obvious issue is the heels lifting from the floor, suggesting short achilles and calf muscles. Less obvious are the flattening of the foot arches that cause the feet to roll inward (overpronation) or the foot rolling outward (underpronation). Ideally, the foot should be in a neutral position.

If, when you do the OHS in front of the mirror, you observe any of these signals with your kinetic chain (the actions and reactions to force that occur in the bones, muscles and nerves whenever dynamic motion or force is required from the body), it really isn't the end of the world. In fact, most people find that they are tight in some areas (if not all of them) when they first try this test. The absolutely fantastic news is that if you do spot any issues, performing the OHS as an exercise, rather than merely a test, will improve your movement pattern, joint range and muscle actions over time.

overhead squat: the results

My rule is that if you cannot perform a perfect OHS, with none of the key warning signs listed above, then you are not ready to perform the power moves in the exercise portfolio. So use the OHS as a guide to whether your body is as ready as your mind is to start doing the toughest, most challenging exercises.

If you find by doing the OHS that your body is not ready, don't think of it as a setback, but rather as a blessing: you are following a training method that is in tune with how the body works, rather than one that merely sets out to punish it.

isolation vs integration

While intensity can be great, when you isolate your muscles you do not get the highly beneficial activity created by the rest of the kinetic chain. I am certainly not saying isolation moves are unproductive, but with the biggest obstacle to exercise being a lack of time, integration work is going to have an instant usable impact on the entire body.

All movements that we do in training or everyday life can be classified as either isolation or integration moves. The vast majority of isolation moves have been created/invented to work specific muscles on their own, with the primary intention of fatiguing that muscle by working it in isolation, usually moving only one joint of the skeleton. Integration, or compound, moves are less of an invention and more of an adaptation of movement patterns that we perform in everyday life. They are designed to work groups of muscles across multiple joints all at the same time.

In real life we never isolate. Even when only a few joints are moving there is a massive number of muscles bracing throughout the body to let the prime muscles do their job. As you go about an average day I doubt you give a second thought to how you are moving. If you take the time to watch the world go by for a few hours, you will notice that human motion consists of just a few combinations of movements that, together, create the millions of potential moves we (hopefully) achieve every day. Everything, and I mean everything, we do boils down to the following key movements:

- Push
- Pull
- Twist
- Squat
- Lunge
- Bend
- Walk
- Run
- Jump

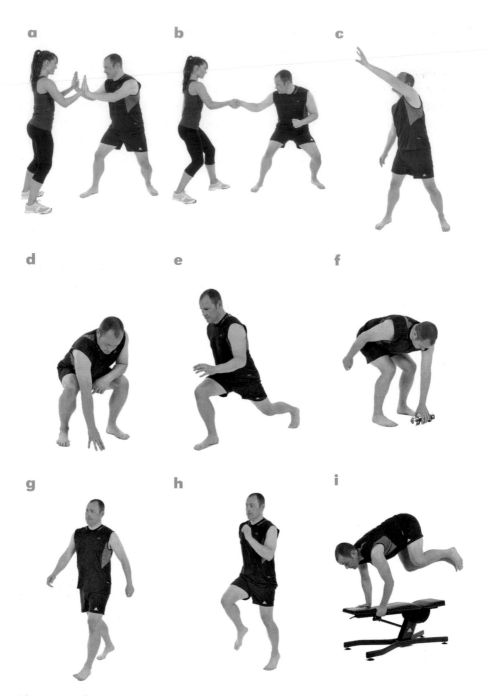

Figure 1 The nine basic human movement patterns: (a) push, (b) pull, (c) twist, (d) squat, (e) lunge, (f) bend, (g) walk, (h) run and (i) jump

All of these movements are integrated. I am certainly not the first person to make this observation, but it constantly amazes me how my industry manages to complicate exercise. With this in mind, I am not a huge fan of old-fashioned machines that isolate small areas of muscle to work them apparently more intensely. While intensity can be great, when you isolate you do not get the highly beneficial activity created by the rest of the kinetic chain. I am certainly not saying isolation moves are unproductive, but with the biggest obstacle to exercise being a lack of time, integration work is going to have an instant usable impact on the entire body.

We would rarely incorporate isolation moves into a workout with a suspension system as this defeats the object of being suspended in the first place. Even when a move is highly targeted towards smaller muscle groups, such as the pecs and the triceps, it would still be considered to be an integration (compound) move because, by being suspended, force is being directed through the lumbopelvic region, which therefore also activates the core stabilisers. Consequently, the majority of the moves in this book are integrated, designed to achieve maximum results in the most economical amount of time.

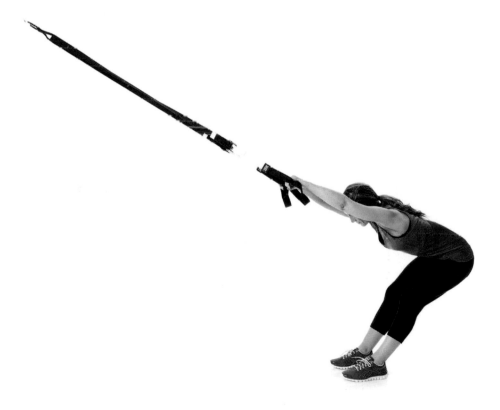

learn it, then work it

As we have discovered, you must walk before you can run in any exercise method, and the body works best if you learn the activity prior to engaging in exercise, so that you will positively soak up the benefits.

Resistance training (using either bodyweight or free weights, or both) is very natural with hardly any complex skills required to achieve results. However, that is not to say you can't get it wrong. In fact, rebuilding the confidence of people who have tried weight training and then failed or injured themselves has featured frequently in my working life. Because of this, I use the phrase 'learn it, then work it' to encourage people to take time to 'imprint' good-quality movement patterns upon their bodies.

how to 'learn it, then work it'

How do you know what 'good-quality' moves look like? Simply put, the move should look smooth and controlled and should not create pain in your joints.

Aim to perform the concentric and eccentric phases (the lift and lower phases) at the same speed – lift for two counts and lower for two counts. When power and speed become more of an objective for you, aim to lift for one count and lower for two counts.

You can perform moves at slower speeds, but that then moves away from how we move/function in day-to-day life; rarely do we do any movement in slow motion just for the sake of it. It is really only beneficial to perform slow or super slow (quarter-speed) moves if you are training for specific sport activities, so as to prolong the time each muscle is under tension (known as 'time under tension'). Therefore, move at a natural speed: athletes and sports people train at 'real time' once they have learned the required movement pattern, so without even knowing it they are 'learning it, then working it'.

The beauty of grounding your workout in the 'learn it, then work it' approach is that by keeping the approach simple, achievable and functional you won't get tied up with methods that either do not work, or have ridiculous expectations of how much time you are going to dedicate to your fitness regime. As a personal trainer, it can be hard to exercise in a gymnasium without wanting to question what many people are (or think they are) doing. So often I see people doing difficult versions of exercises that are clearly beyond their level of ability – presumably because they think difficult/advanced must equal quicker results. The obvious signs are that they can't control the weights or their body seems overpowered by the movements it is being asked to do. 'Learn it, then work it' relates to most physical tasks in life, but especially sport; for example, if you have tennis lessons, the first thing you would learn would be to make contact with the ball slowly rather than starting with the fastest, hardest movements. So simply switch off your instincts to 'work hard' until you are satisfied that you can move and maintain quality and control throughout the repetition.

As you get more adventurous and diverse with your exercise remember that all your goals are achievable: if you're moving, you're improving.

'learn it, then work it' in sport

Practising movements in resistance training is paralleled in all performance-based sports. Athletes routinely perform low intensity 'drills', which echo the moves they need to make in their sport. For example, during almost every track session, sprinters practise knee lifts, heel flicks and other bounding exercises to improve their quality of movement and condition their muscles in a highly functional manner.

first you need stability

Stability is the first key ingredient to ensure safe and effective exercise; the basic building block for everything that follows in this book.

To perform exercise safely and effectively, we first have to ensure our body is stable. The essence of stability is the ability to control and transfer force throughout the body. All human movement is, in fact, a chain of events involving the brain, the nervous system, muscles, fascia, ligaments and tendons. So, while a simple move like a bicep curl may appear to involve only activity from the shoulder down to the hand, in reality there is a chain of events that occur to ensure that the right amount of force is applied and that the two ends of the bicep are tethered to a stable base.

In essence, wherever there is visible movement in the body, there are always invisible reactions occurring within the kinetic chain to facilitate this movement.

The engine room of all this activity is in the deep muscles of the trunk, specifically:

- transversus abdominus (TA);
- multifidi (MF);
- internal obliques;
- five layers of muscle and fascia that make up the pelvic floor.

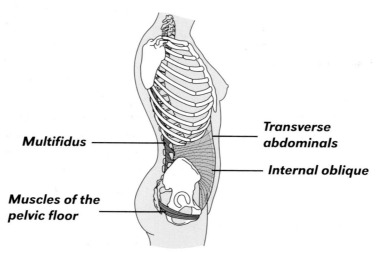

Figure 2 The deep muscles of the trunk are crucial for stability

These muscles work as a team and their simultaneous contraction is known as 'co-contraction'. This complex muscle activity produces intra-abdominal pressure (IAP) and it is the creation of this pressure that stabilises the lumbar spine. The misconception that the transversus abdominus looks like a 'belt' around the torso no doubt led fitness instructors to continually advise clients to pull their stomach in (hollow the abdominal muscles), thinking that this would amplify the stability of the spine. However, it is not simply the recruitment of these muscles that instils strength and stability, but, more importantly, when they are recruited. In effect, they should have been advising clients to 'switch on' (brace their core).

remember: don't hollow your abs

Pulling in, or hollowing, the abs actually makes you less able to stabilise. If you imagine a tree that is perfectly vertical, but then you chop in or hollow out one side, the structure of the tree becomes less stable. I have two ways of coaching the correct technique to avoid hollowing the abs, depending on the client:

1 Switch on your abs as if you were going to get punched in the stomach; or
2 Engage the abs in the same way as if you were about to be tickled.

Both methods achieve the desired outcome – with only a few of my male clients insisting that I really do hit them!

Stability is, therefore, a goal in everything that we do. However, we shouldn't have to undertake yet more training just to achieve core stability; rather, we should ensure that the everyday movements we make encourage the muscles deep inside the trunk to work correctly during dynamic movements, and that the stabilisation is instinctive, as opposed to something that we have to remind ourselves to do every time. For instance, if you drop an egg in the kitchen and very quickly squat and make a grab to catch it, you don't stop to think or choreograph the movement. Your body will have fired off a co-contraction which enabled you to grab the egg before it hit the ground (or, at least, make a good attempt). When I use this analogy to explain the concept of stability to my clients, they often get a twinkle in their eye, for if this process is instinctive, why should they continue to train? The reality, however, is that you still have to exercise that instinct to keep the system working properly: 'use it, or lose it'.

In the workout sessions later in this book, you will find that almost all the moves are classified as being good for stability. Since stability is the first stage of development, you might assume the strength and power moves that follow are more productive because they are more 'intense'. While this is true, that intensity will only be constructive if the body has the ability to control and direct all that extra force, which can only be learned through the stability moves.

the development of core stability in the fitness industry

During the 1990s, there were only three components of fitness that personal trainers focused on with the average client (by 'average' I mean a person looking for fitness gains rather than to compete in sport). Cardio was the route to cardiovascular efficiency and was the most obvious tool for weight loss; strength training isolated the larger muscle groups and gymnasiums were filled with straight line machines; and we only worked on flexibility because we knew we had to, but the chosen method was predominantly the least productive type of stretching, i.e. static.

Then, it seems almost from nowhere, there was a new ingredient to every workout: core stability. New equipment such as Swiss balls and modern versions of wobble boards, such as the Reebok Core Board® and the BOSU® (Both Sides Up), increased the wave of enthusiasm for this type of training as, of course, did the new popularity for the more physical versions of yoga and Pilates.

In retrospect, we in the fitness industry could have thought to ourselves that we had been doing everything wrong up to that point. However, the reality is that rather than being 'wrong' we were just learning as we went along. In fact, many of the methods that suddenly became mainstream had been used in sports training for years before, but without the 'label' of core stability, and rather than treating them as an individual component, we trained them instinctively as part of our dynamic strength moves using bodyweight or free weights.

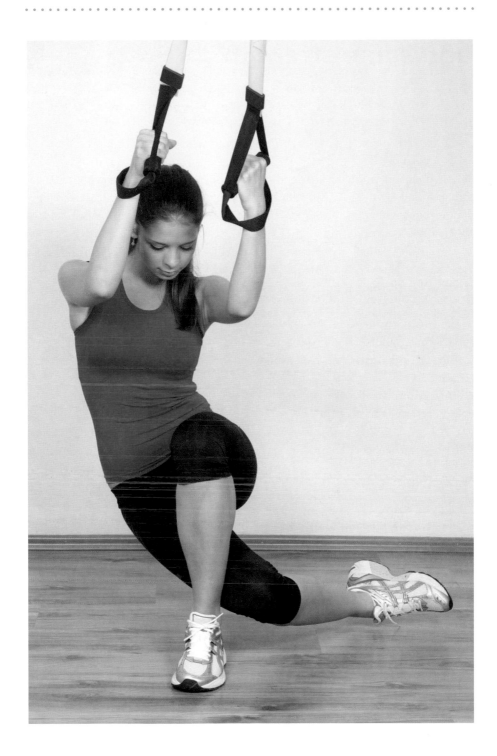

add some strength

The second key ingredient. There are several types of strength that you can gain performing these exercises – strength endurance, elastic strength and maximum strength.

When trying to establish a client's fitness objectives, 'I want to improve my strength' is often the only information given to a personal trainer. This seemingly simple request requires much more detail if you are going to achieve the outcome that is really desired.

The one-line definition of strength is: 'An ability to exert a physical force against resistance'. However, this catch-all is not specific enough when you are dealing with strength. In fact, there are three main types of strength:

1 **Strength endurance**: Achieved when you aim to exert force many times in close succession.
2 **Elastic strength**: Achieved when you make fast contractions to change position.
3 **Maximum strength**: Our ability over a single repetition to generate our greatest amount of force.

Each of these specific types of strength can be achieved using resistance, either as individual components or (preferably) as part of an integrated approach.

Unless you are an athlete training for an event that requires a disproportionate amount of either endurance, elastic or maximum strength, then the integration of functional training methods will create a body that is more designed to cope with day-to-day life and amateur sports. While strength is an adaptation that the body willingly accepts, the reality is that changes take time, so treat strength gains as something that happens over weeks, months and years rather than mere days.

power and speed come with practice

The development of power in muscles is a rapid process and is also considerably practical, usable and functional for those men and women who have reached a point in their training where they don't need to be any 'stronger', but they want to make more of the strength they have.

Power is a measure of how much energy is created, the amount of force applied and the velocity at which it is applied. It is the ability to exert an explosive burst of movement. In everyday life it presents as bounding up stairs three at a time or pushing a heavy weight above your head. The development of power is not only a more rapid process than developing maximal strength, but is also considerably more practical, usable and functional for those men and women who have reached a point in their training where they have no desire to be any 'stronger', but they do want to make more of the strength they have. That is the point at which you stop thinking about increasing the amount of resistance you work against and start thinking about how to inject speed into the activity you are doing with your suspension system.

Let's make this simple. If you have two men of the same height, weight and with the same body fat levels and you challenge them to compete against each other in an explosive activity that they have both trained in, such as a 20m sprint, then, apart from potential differences in reaction times, the man who wins that race will be the one who has a greater ability to utilise his strength and convert that strength into forward motion. This ability to use strength for explosive activity is power. The perfect exercise to generate this type of outcome would be the squat against a wall with a jump as this move trains you to generate an explosive force that propels the body quickly.

When you get to the exercises in the portfolio classified as power moves, you will see that they are in fact progressions of the skills that you will have already developed during your stability and strength sessions, but performed at speed. In this respect, it becomes easier to understand why I advise not to skip a stage when learning movement patterns ('learn it, then work it').

To train or develop power using predominately bodyweight exercises with a suspension system is realistic, but only as long as you do not get preoccupied with the speed part of the equation to the detriment of working against resistance. It is very easy to 'cheat' (or under-perform) with a suspension system as the intensity has an infinite number of easily adjusted variables – cheating/under-performing can be classed as not doing a full range of motion, shifting your bodyweight so that the exercise becomes easier or simply not putting any force against the touch-points (your torso, hands and feet) – any of these 'cheating tactics' will allow you to move faster but you will probably not be using as much strength as you would without the adaptation.

power and agility

Think of power as a very close relation of agility; you don't learn agility by overloading and working while fatigued – rather you develop it by achieving quality over quantity. In fact, introducing yourself to the pursuit of power can mean performing the moves without any weights and simply performing the movements fast with just bodyweight as the resistance. Why? Because athletic power is actually a finely tuned combination of speed and strength.

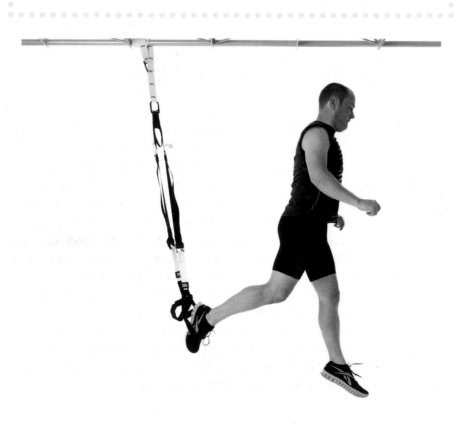

2 the portfolio of moves

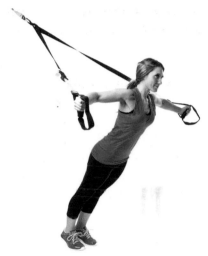

which moves should I do?

This section contains a portfolio of moves that I have selected from those I use every day with my personal training clients and are based on the principles I explained in the first part of this book. The only moves that have made it into this book are those that deserve to be here – every one of these moves is tried and tested to ensure it gets results; in fact, I have spent hundreds of hours using them myself and thousands of hours teaching them to my personal training clients, who over the years have included men and women from 16 to 86 years old, from size zero through to 280lbs. These clients have, justifiably, only been interested in the moves that work – and these are what you have here in this portfolio.

It is not an exhaustive list of moves, simply because many extra moves that could have been included use a suspension system simply as a 'prop' rather than a tool, or they are really just subtle adaptations of those included here. For instance, changes to foot position and the amount of bend that you have in your arms and legs will encourage the body to recruit slightly different muscles, but I would class these as adaptations rather than unique moves.

presentation of the moves

I wanted to show the moves as a complete portfolio, rather than simply wrapping them up into workouts, because you are then able to see how the stability, strength and power versions relate to each other. Understanding these progressions is something I encourage in my clients because they need to know that subtle changes can make all the difference between a good use of time and a waste of it. By thinking this way you can very quickly learn all the moves because, in the majority of cases, the main movement pattern stays the same throughout the stability, strength and power progressions, with only a slight change to the length of levers (arm/foot positions), range of motion or the speed.

crazy stuff...

There will always be those people who will try to dream up moves with products like a suspension system that are either dangerous, pointless, or just plain stupid. The gym ball seems to attract these people more than any other item of equipment – I see people standing on balls, diving on balls, hitting balls and generally abusing themselves or the product. Just because you can do something on a ball doesn't mean that it is productive or safe. Fortunately, suspension systems don't seem to have fallen victim to this treatment in the same way.

In my other books I have included a section called 'Trash – don't waste your time'. However, with this book when I started doing my research I realised that while I had witnessed plenty of crazy, tough and often bizarre exercises being performed with suspension systems, most of them were justifiable as long as they were being performed by individuals that had reached a very high level of competence in both skill and physical ability. However, there are still general uses that I think are more about showing off than actually having a productive value so they have ended up in the section called 'Crazy stuff I won't ask you to do' (see page 108).

The third part of this book goes on to present a selection of training sessions, designed for a range of levels, and following my method of progressing through stability, strength and power exercises. No doubt some people will jump straight to the training sessions; however, I find understanding the 'why' as well as knowing the 'how' generates better outcomes for most people, so refer back to the portfolio of moves if you want the detailed description of how to perform the exercise. I have also provided you with a post-workout stretch session suitable for all types of resistance training (see pages 115–118). Please remember that you should always warm up before embarking on any type of exercise.

every muscle plays a part

I purposefully haven't included diagrams of the muscles that are targeted by each move as hopefully by now you understand that, used correctly, every muscle plays a role in every move.

I have written the descriptions as if I am talking to you as a client – the key information for each explanation includes:

- the correct body position at the start and end of the move;
- the movement that you are looking to create.

When I work with my PT clients I avoid over-coaching the movement as my goal is to see them move in a lovely 'fluid' way, where the whole movement blends together.

reps
This is a 'learn it' section rather than 'work it'. Therefore, for the vast majority of the moves I don't talk about how many repetitions you should do of each – that information is included in the workout section in the third part of the book. How many repetitions you perform should relate to your objectives; almost all the moves can be used to improve stability, strength and power (at the same time), and the speed and resistance at which you perform it will dictate the outcome. For example, a slow squat performed with a light weight will provide stability benefits. Exactly the same move performed with a heavier weight will increase strength, and the same move at speed will develop power.

intensity
Exercise with a suspension system creates a unique situation in terms of how intensity can be 'adjusted' or manipulated. On page 17 I describe how your body position in relation to the anchor point changes the challenge to your muscles and energy systems. Both the position of your hands and feet and the angle of your body is going to affect your ability to complete the target time/repetitions on each exercise so make sure that you have practised all the moves and become familiar with how to make quick subtle changes to your body position mid set.

tricks of the trade

For each exercise, I have included a 'tricks of the trade' box which contains a nugget of information that I use to help my clients get the most out of each exercise.

key to exercises

As you move through the exercises, you will notice that each is identified by the following key words. A quick glance will tell you which element the move focuses on, what type of move it is and whether you need any additional equipment to perform it.

stability

Every move in this portfolio is a stability-enhancing exercise. Yes, that includes the strength and power versions. Stability is, essentially, a reaction within the kinetic chain in which the body says to itself: 'Switch on the muscles around the lumbopelvic region, because this movement is looking for an anchor point to latch on to'. On this basis, you don't improve stability when you are sat down on a solid surface, but you do when sitting on a gym ball, standing on a wobble board and in the majority of cases when 'supported' on a suspension system. Likewise you generally won't improve stability when a move only involves one joint.

strength

We could get all deep and meaningful about biomechanics here, but to qualify as a strength move, the exercise needs to be making you move a force through space using muscle contractions. Therefore, anything that only involves momentum is a waste of time because you are just going along for the ride and not actively contracting your muscles. However, don't confuse speed with momentum – speed is good, especially when mixed with strength, because that combination develops the highly desirable power.

power

Every time you read the word 'power' you need to think of speed, and vice versa. The maths and physics required to understand how we measure power are enough to make you glaze over, and in reality you are much better off measuring your power ability by doing a simple time-trial sprint, or timing yourself over a set number of repetitions, rather than trying to calculate exactly how much power you are exerting for a specific exercise.

If you want more power, you need to move fast, but you need to be able to maintain speed while pushing or pulling a weight (that weight could be an object or your own body). For example, you might have a guy who can skip across a shot-put circle faster than the other guy when not holding and throwing the shot, but he is only speedy. The guy who can move fast and launch the shot (using strength) is the one with all the power.

suspended stretches

I have two different modes when I stretch:

1 If I am actively trying to increase my flexibility (stretch mode), I take the position to the point of discomfort, hold it then keep going a little further. When the muscle relaxes, I release the stretch for a moment then go back into the stretch position again – the minimum time I spend doing this is 30 seconds per stretch. There's no upper limit on how long you can stretch for, although it is essential that you do all the stretches equally rather than just focusing on the ones you enjoy or find easy.

2 When I am chilled out (relax mode), I just get into positions that are comfortable and enjoy the moment.

The following stretches are a combination of both. There are many other stretches that you can use, but I find that many of them incorporate the suspension system for the sake of it, and that you are often better off doing a similar stretch on the floor. This selection uses the suspension system to enhance the stretch, rather than just using it as an accessory.

When doing any of the workouts I suggest doing all of these stretches at the end of the session (see pages 115–118).

- Suspended hip stretch
- Supported inner thigh
- Suspended 'C' stretch
- Supported back extension
- Supported down dog

dynamic warm-up moves

exercise 1 upper back dynamic stretch

● **prepares body**   **strap length: medium**

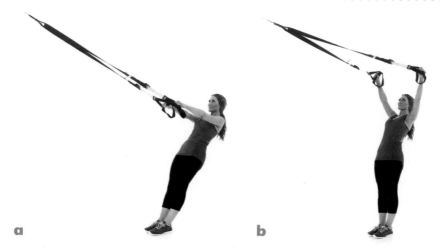

a   b

Getting a movement just right has a name – 'instinct'. This is when everything just falls into place and happens perfectly. Athletes achieve this by performing drills which are in effect small parts of the desired movement. Each of these warm-up moves plays a role in the 'big picture' of movement quality, so never skip the warm-up.

● Stand with your feet together, the straps should be tight, but the level of intensity should feel easy.
● Lean back with straight arms and round your shoulders.
● Lift your arms straight up in front of you while at the same time squeezing your shoulder blades together

tricks of the trade
Take a really big, chest-expanding breath when stretching to mobilise the rib cage – it will make you feel strong inside.

exercise 2 dynamic chest stretch

• prepares body   **strap length: medium**

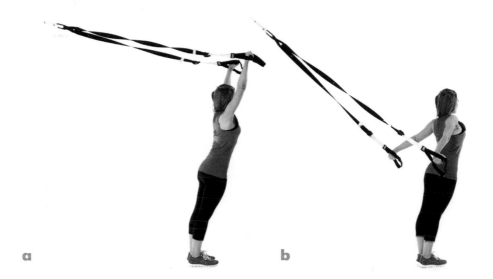

a   b

For a muscle to be able to exert its full potential of available force, the joint it passes over must move freely. With new clients (especially desk workers), I often find that their range of motion is awful, in particular around the shoulders and upper back. So, while they think they should be thrashing around 'working out', the reality is they need to master the warm-up moves first.

- With your feet together, extend your arms behind you and take up the slack in the straps.
- Transfer your weight on and off the front leg and let your arms be gently pulled behind you.

tricks of the trade

I want you to 'creep up' on this move rather than forcing it. If you are tight in this area, improving mobility could improve everything from your breathing to your bench press.

exercise 3 low back dynamic stretch

● **prepares body**   **strap length: medium**

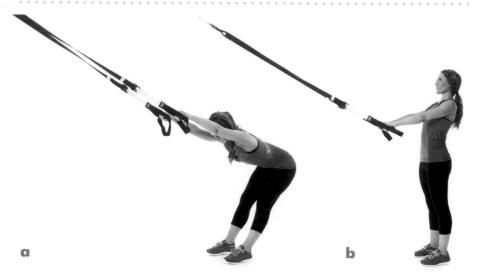

a   b

With many suspension moves 'switching on' the core (something isolation moves fail to do), it is essential to bring the pelvis and lower back joint complex into action early on in every suspension workout. If you still need convincing, just try this move and you'll experience how fantastic it feels.

● Hold the handles and step away from the anchor until the straps are tight.
● Bend forward (hip hinge) and at the same time let your hips drop backwards.
● Look to create a '>' shape with your body and move in and out of the pose – this feels fantastic on the hamstring muscles and lower back.

> ## tricks of the trade
> When in the suspended position, try rotating your hands so you feel the stretch in different parts of your shoulders.

exercise 4 torso shoulder rotation

● **prepares body**   **strap length: medium**

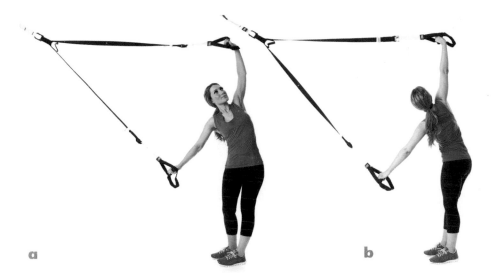

a   b

'Never have any slack in your strap' is a good mantra to have when using your suspension system. As you perform this warm-up exercise, there is a temptation to simply wave your arms around; however, if you can keep the strap tight and move your feet and body, you will get a vastly improved 'connection' between you and the resistance.

● Hold both handles at waist height and stand with your feet shoulder-width apart.
● Letting the suspension system take your weight, rotate your torso while taking one arm high and the other low.
● Swing in the other direction quickly but with control.

tricks of the trade
This move needn't look too 'perfect', so keep it relaxed and focus on making the move flow.

exercise 5 little jumps

● **prepares body**   **strap length: medium**

a   b

For an exercise to be functional it needn't resemble something you do in your everyday life. This is why I sometimes prefer the term 'transferable skills' to the word 'functional'. This move is one such example: if you break down the individual components of it, there are some fantastic neuro and physical triggers involved.

● Hold the handles at chest height and lean away from the anchor point.
● Jump your feet apart to shoulder-width quickly.
● Keep the knees slightly bent on landing, then jump your feet back together. The jumps should be light and bouncy.

tricks of the trade
While this is in the warm-up list, there is no reason you can't also use this as an energy blast between strength moves.

strength and conditioning

exercise 6 row

● **stability** ● **strength**   **strap length: medium**

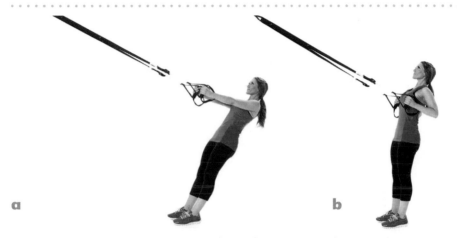

a   b

This is invariably the first exercise we all try when we get our hands on a suspension system. And we all fit into two categories of people: those who stand up straight and ask what all the fuss is about; and those that lay flat with their feet directly under the anchor point and swing all over the place. Calm down – this is a great move but you should take some time to get your level right as it will be a similar scenario with a lot of the other moves.

● Hold the grips, take up the slack and position your feet in the appropriate position (based on the Suspension Spiral – see page 16).
● Start with straight arms and pull your body towards the handles and then slowly release.
● Aim to squeeze your shoulder blades together, but avoid shrugging your shoulders.

tricks of the trade
Look above the anchor point: this will encourage you to retract your scapula (shoulder blade).

exercise 7 chest press

● stability ● strength   strap length: medium

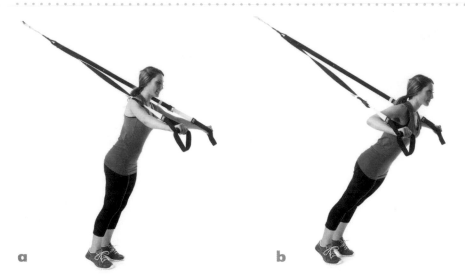

a   b

Nine times out of ten the straps will rub on your forearms when you first do this move – it's not right but it isn't the end of the world. Getting into the correct position takes practice and when working out with suspension systems, you'll also notice that almost every time you use them you can have a different experience.

● Stand and lean forwards so that the straps take your weight. Keep a space between your forearms and the straps.
● Bend your elbows and widen your hand position as your body moves towards the floor.
● When your chest is level with your hands, push against the handles to drive your body back to the start position.

tricks of the trade
If the straps rub on your forearms, push outwards instead of straight in front of you. This will stop the rub and also hit the pecs harder.

exercise 8 squat

● stability ● strength   **strap length: medium**

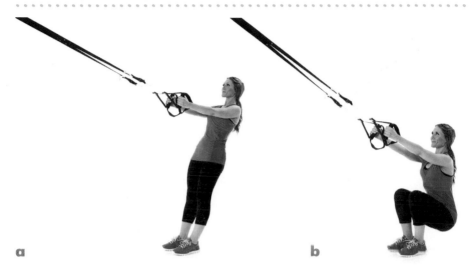

a   b

It is very easy for bad technique to creep into a regular squat (heels lifting, bowing forwards, etc.), but when you are suspended all those transgressions are smoothed out. Admittedly some of your total bodyweight is supported by the straps, but that small negative is outweighed for many people by their sudden ability to squat like a baby (deep with the knees behind the toes).

● Step away from the anchor until the straps are tight and your arms are at shoulder height.
● Look up at the anchor point. Your weight should be spread evenly across the front and back of your foot.
● Squat down (don't pull on the suspension system, just let it take some of your weight).
● When you can't squat any lower, stand back up. You will most likely feel your weight shift into your heels on the way up.

tricks of the trade

The number-one challenge here can simply be gripping the floor! The solution is to squeeze your inner thigh muscles together slightly and you will feel more grounded (but don't let your knees touch).

exercise 9 back extension

● **stability** ● **strength**   **strap length: medium**

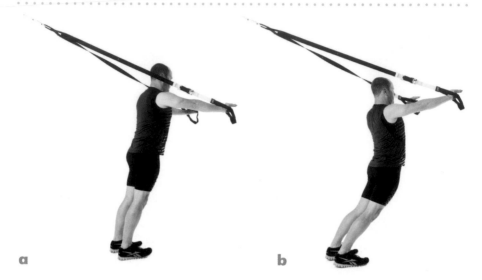

a   b

Some moves have subtle requirements. This one can so easily turn into a shoulder exercise if you 'relax' through your shoulders – but the clue to getting it right is in the name. In the 'release' phase of the exercise, when you are extending, it's easy to just 'let go', but avoid this and make the concentric and eccentric timing equal.

● Hold the grips, take up the slack and position your feet in the appropriate position (based on the Suspension Spiral).
● The joints in your arms, shoulder and chest stay fixed throughout this movement.
● Keep a straight line from your hip, knee and ankle and extend backwards with your spine. This move feels very powerful if you can keep all the fixed areas locked.

tricks of the trade
Breathe out as you extend. Held breath creates a 'solid' void inside you and will restrict your range of motion.

exercise 10 bicep curl

• stability • strength   **strap length: medium**

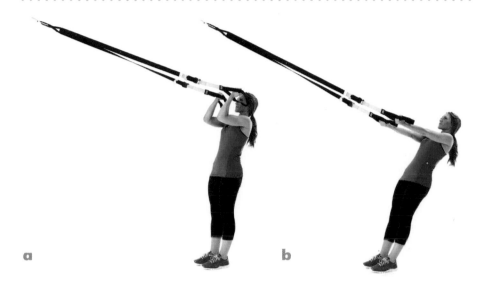

a   b

When is a bicep curl not a bicep curl? When you are on a suspension system. Body angle and foot position can transform this isolation move (one of the few you can do with a suspension system). Being suspended transforms this humble curl into a completely different, whole-body experience.

- Let the suspension support your bodyweight and raise your arms in front to shoulder height.
- Your hands should stay shoulder-width apart.
- Aim to keep a straight line from your shoulder down to hip, knee and ankle.
- Curl your arms towards you until your hands reach the sides of your face, then slowly uncurl your arms.

tricks of the trade

It's absolutely fine to separate your elbows slightly. You'll still be targeting the biceps, but at the same time you will find it more comfortable.

exercise 11 side lunge

● stability ● strength   **strap length: medium**

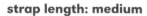

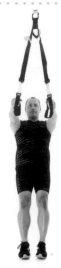
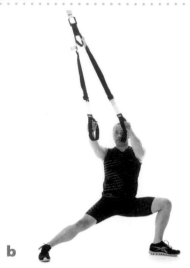

a   b

When you have been using a product for a long time (I first tried suspension exercise in 2007), it's always interesting to see and hear the reaction from people experiencing it for the first time. Interestingly with some of the suspension leg exercises they say 'suspension makes them easier'. Well, yes and no. In fact, it doesn't make them easier, just different – your body still weighs the same as when you do a regular lunge, but here the weight is spread between more touch-points.

● If you stand too close to the anchor, this move changes its characteristics – so concentrate on the width of your lunge rather than a smaller V/F angle.
● Lean back standing with your feet together. The arm position stays high and long.
● Step outwards. The stepping foot turns out at almost 90 degrees, while the supporting foot remains pointing at the anchor point.

> **tricks of the trade**
> Try not to punctuate this movement so let one repetition flow into the next and don't pause in the middle – go straight onto the next leg.

exercise 12 triceps press

● stability ● strength   **strap length: medium**

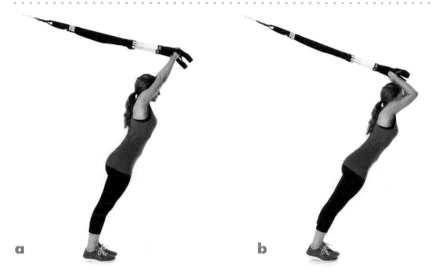

a   b

This move becomes a beast of an exercise when you get your body past 45 degrees, while at the same time it becomes super simple if you are fairly upright. Subtle changes to where and how you hold the handle will call into action more than just the triceps. Some might call this cheating but frankly that's nonsense as we really aren't trying to isolate but to comprehensibly integrate as many muscle reactions as we can – if you are moving, you are improving!

● Raise your arms above your head, keeping your body straight. With your hands shoulder-width apart, lean forwards so the straps support your bodyweight.
● As your arms bend, your tricep muscles will be taking more of your weight. Keep the eccentric contraction going until until your elbows are at full range.
● Press hard against the handles (at this point your core will react to the change of direction), and keep pressing until your arms are straight and then repeat.

tricks of the trade
I find it really natural to do a calf raise during this move. I know it's supposed to be a triceps exercise but with suspension exercise I think we are better off thinking 'all muscles all of the time'.

exercise 13 prone plank on elbows

● stability ● strength   **strap length: long**

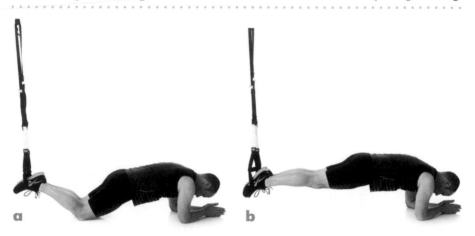

a   b

For the first ten years of my fitness career, there were no 'planks'. Then along came the resurgence of Pilates and they were everywhere. I remember things getting a little ridiculous when in a class we held the plank for as long as possible and a gorgeous lady called Nicky held it for over four minutes – that's impressive but sadly of little practical use. Thankfully the addition of a suspension system turns this static challenge into a dynamic tussle between the straps and your touch-points.

● Hook your feet over the foot straps, lay on your front and keep your feet slightly apart.
● Your elbows should be touching your ribs at the start of the move. Your shoulders stay at the same height throughout the exercise.
● Lift your hips, thighs and abs off the floor until your shoulder, hip, knee and ankle are all in a straight line.
● Pause in the raised position for 2–3 seconds, then slowly return to the floor and repeat.

tricks of the trade

Try to do one complete breathing cycle (breathe in and out) in the raised position – your lungs and diaphragm play a massive role in core/torso stabilisation.

exercise 14 supine plank

● stability ● strength   **strap length: long**

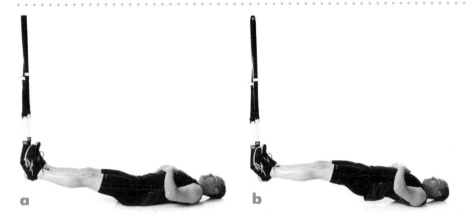

a   b

Firstly, this is not a neck exercise so please avoid the most common mistake which is to tilt the head back, giving the impression that you have moved a lot when in fact you are just looking behind you. Secondly, have faith in the heel straps; your bodyweight pressing down on them should be enough to keep your feet in place (have them resting on the back of your heels rather than directly on your Achilles tendon).

● Place your feet in the foot straps while directly under the anchor point, then shuffle your body backwards. Be aware that moving only a small distance backwards (as shown in picture b) increases the intensity of the exercise significantly.
● Support your upper body on your elbows and forearms, then lift your hips up. Your touch-points are the heels, hands, forearms and shoulders.
● Pause in the raised position for 2 3 seconds, then slowly return to the floor and repeat.

tricks of the trade

Look at the anchor point throughout this move or you may make the common mistake of throwing your head back as you lift your hips.

exercise 15 balance lunge

● stability ● strength   **strap length: medium**

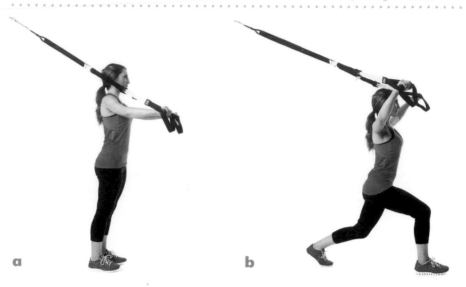

a   b

This move verges on being a single leg lunge, which is one of the most worthwhile exercises to master for all-round low back, hip and leg conditioning. When holding the straps remember the mantra 'no slack in the straps' and actively push your weight into the handles.

● Stand with your feet halfway between the anchor point and handles.
● Press your weight into the handles and step forwards so that your foot goes ahead of the handles.
● Then, while maintaining pressure on the handles, return to the start position.

!

tricks of the trade
Avoid having the straps touch your torso and note that taking your hands wider will increase muscle activity in your upper body without detracting from the lower body work.

exercise 16 suspended bridge

• stability • strength   **strap length: long**

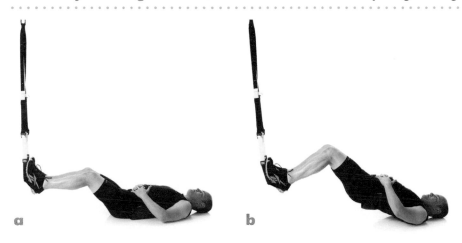

a   b

This is definitely a move that I class as a 'demo' move as I would always use it to quickly get clients to understand the principles and benefits of being suspended. Once you get comfortable with the foot position and realise that your feet won't fall out, you can start to get more daylight under your lower back and glutes – then when you are ready, go 'hands free' (as in photos above).

- Place your feet in the foot straps while directly under the anchor point, then shuffle your body backwards.
- Lift your hips up. Your touch-points are the heels, hands and shoulders (avoid pressing your head hard against the floor).
- Pause in the raised position for 2–3 seconds, then slowly return to the floor and repeat.

> **! tricks of the trade**
>
> Don't let your knees, feet or ankles touch each other. This will make the move slightly harder, but give you much greater core strength and balance gains.

exercise 17 hamstring curl

● stability ● strength   **strap length: long**

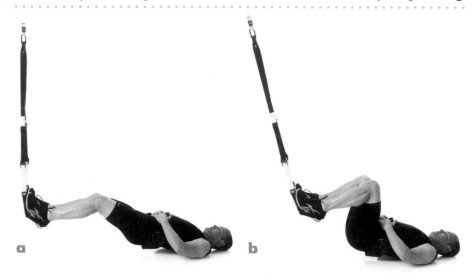

a   b

We aren't looking to isolate muscles during suspension system training, but rather integrate them. However, with this move, you will definitely feel that your hamstrings and glutes are dominant – without doubt this move promotes the reaction of 'wow I can really feel that'.

● Place your feet in the foot straps while directly under the anchor point, then shuffle your body backwards.
● Lift your hips up. Your touch points are the heels and shoulders (again, avoid pressing your head hard against the floor).
● Bend your knees until your heels are as close to your glutes as possible then lengthen the legs again and repeat.

tricks of the trade

Confession time: some people get cramp the first time they do this move! It won't cause you any damage, but can be a bit of a shock, so just straighten your leg until it goes, then start again.

exercise 18 lunge step back

● stability ● strength   **strap length: medium**

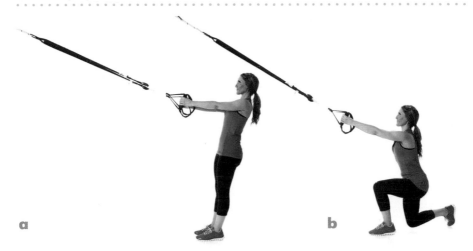

a   b

This move is a prime candidate for half measures – it's just too easy to stand and hold the handle then step back. So before you even think about lunging, step right back until you have straps held above chest or even shoulder height – now you are ready.

● Most of the work is done with the front leg rather than the leg that travels back into the lunge, so keep focused on the front leg's position.
● Step back keeping the straps long and tight then repeat on the other leg.
● It's very tempting to pull with your arms but resist this as much as possible.

tricks of the trade
The suspension system should give you the confidence to lunge really deeply so don't feel that using the straps to pull against is cheating – the attitude should be 'every muscle every rep'.

exercise 19 squat, back to anchor

● stability ● strength   **strap length: medium**

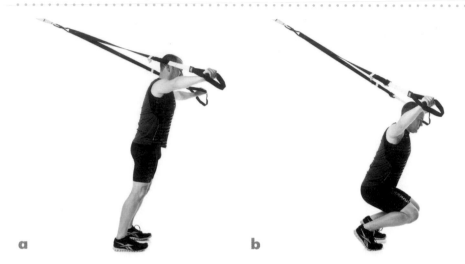

a   b

New personal trainers often fall into the habit of applying the same rules to every exercise that they do. For example, on most squats I would encourage you to keep the heels touching the floor, but if I demanded that on this move, I would find that very few people could actually do it – and the only way I know this is because I don't ask anybody to do anything I haven't tried myself (too many personal trainers don't abide by this rule).

● Lean forwards until you are between 70 and 45 degrees V/F angle. Your weight will be on the front of your feet and your core will be active.
● Squat down until you reach at least a 90 degree angle at the knee. During this part of the exercise your heels lift off the floor.
● As you squat, the handles and straps will travel up and down parallel to the depth of your squat.

tricks of the trade

This move should never get boring; if you need to spice it up, try turning your feet inwards for half the reps and then outwards for the other half (approx 15 degrees in and out).

exercise 20 hip dip

● **stability** ● **strength**   **strap length: short/medium**

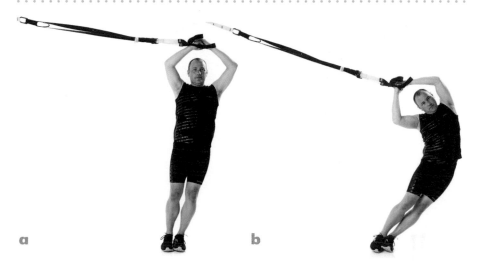

a   b

This is another 'wow' exercise. You will find that every time you do it you need to adjust your feet towards the anchor point slightly to ensure that you can feel it working through your waist and into the outside of your ribcage. Keep the move slow; otherwise it tends to become a bit of a bounce rather than a transition from eccentric to concentric.

● Step away from the vertical axis but stay standing upright. Hold your arms above your head (forming a circle), but don't let your arms touch the side of your head yet.
● Drop your hip away from the anchor and as you bend at the waist you should try to make your head touch your bicep (the side furthest from the anchor).
● Engage the muscles in your waist to pull you back into the start position.

tricks of the trade

Avoid pushing your hips forwards or back during this move – imagine you are sandwiched between two panes of glass that you must not touch!

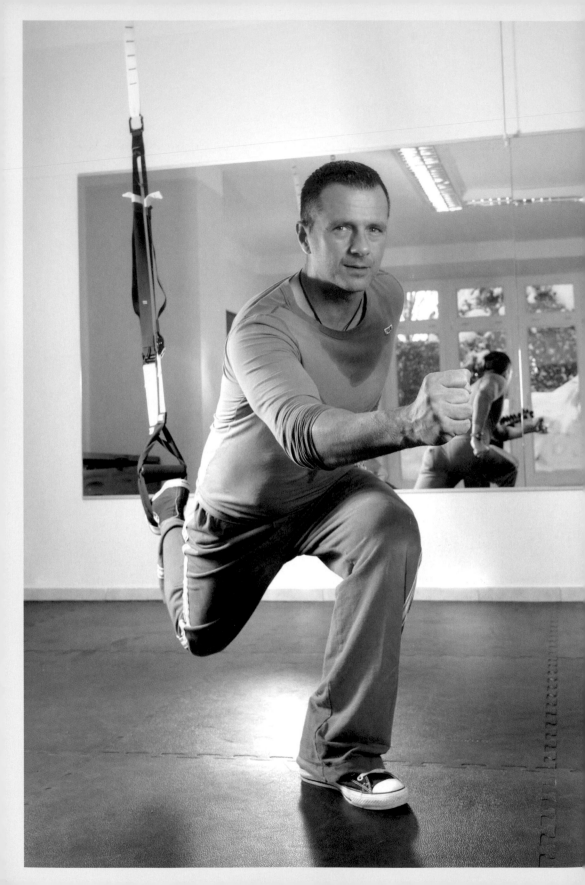

exercise 21 y fly

● **stability** ● **strength**　　　　　　　　　　**strap length: medium**

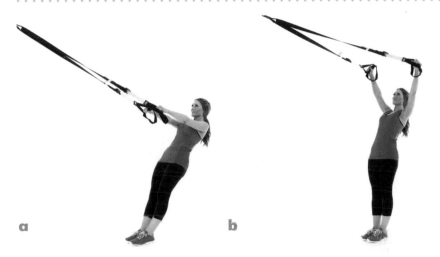

a　　　　　　　　　　　b

The sensation that you enjoy during this move is really quite interesting. If you perform a similar movement with dumbbells, the weight becomes 'weightless' when you reach the top of the movement – but when you reach full range with suspension straps, the pause at the top remains very switched on, especially if you rock back on your heels a little.

● Start in a 45 degree V/F angle with your arms straight. The only obvious joints that should move are the shoulders.
● Engage the muscles in your upper back and shoulders by raising your arms high and wide.
● When your torso is just off vertical and hands are at their highest, pause and slowly fold your body forwards back into the start position.

tricks of the trade
Aim to keep your hand, wrist and forearms all in line with each other. This will build your grip strength which is key to getting better at many of the other upper body moves.

exercise 22 overhead squat, facing anchor

● stability ● strength   **strap length: medium**

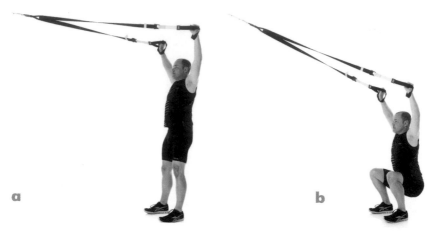

a   b

The overhead squat is one of my favourite moves already, so the addition of an extra touch-point in the hands makes it remarkable. This time I do want the heels to stay in contact with the floor; in fact I want you to 'go light' on the balls of your feet and tease the suspension straps to take as much weight as you can exert on them while keeping your arms and shoulders pulled back.

● With your arms raised above your head, step away from the anchor point until the straps are tight. Now, take a small step towards the anchor point (so your feet are slightly in front of your hands and the straps are supporting your weight).
● Look up at the anchor point. Your weight should be spread evenly across the front and back of your foot.
● Squat down, but don't pull on the suspension system, just let it take some of your weight.
● When you can't squat any lower, stand back up (you will most likely feel your weight shift into your heels on the way up).

tricks of the trade

This is one of the moves that is more than the sum of its parts. That's why I use a version of it to test for the quality of movement in all my clients, so 'practise, practise, practise' as it will be time well spent.

exercise 23 overhead squat, back to anchor

● **stability** ● **strength**   **strap length: medium**

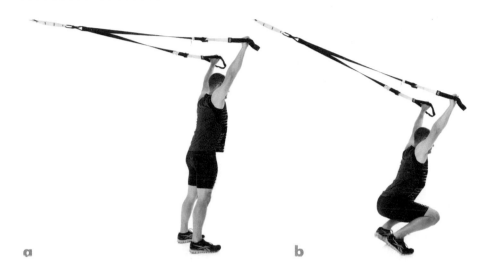

a   b

This is harder than it looks so please stick with it. Your heels will be lifted and the muscle activation should be very obvious in every muscle between your hands and feet. Feel free to take your feet closer to the anchor after a few reps but not if this causes any slack in the straps (that's cheating).

● Lean forwards until you are between 70 and 45 degrees V/F angle.
● Your heels will lift off the floor as soon as you start to squat down and your core will be engaged to enable you to keep your arms raised straight above your head.
● Squat down until you reach at least a 90 degree angle at the knees, then stand back up.

tricks of the trade
As you squat, the handles and straps should travel up and down parallel to the depth of your squat. If they don't, you don't have your shoulders fixed in place as well as you should have!

75

exercise 24 x fly

● **stability** ● **strength**   **strap length: medium**

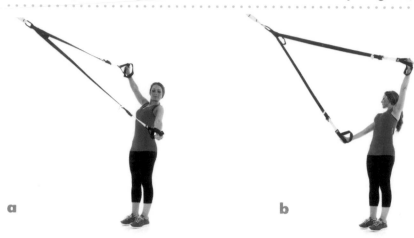

a   b

There was a time when almost everything we did in gymnasiums was perfectly symmetrical, but not any more. I call this move the X fly because the aim is to create an '/' shape when your right arm is raised and then an '\' shape when the left arm is raised, putting those two together creates an X hence the name. Keep your arms very straight throughout this move – if you bend your elbows, you will lose much of the impact.

● Load the suspension straps by leaning back between 30 and 45 degrees V/F. Your arms should be in front of you at chest height.
● Using just the muscles in your shoulders and upper back, drive one arm up and the other down towards your hip. Most of the work is done when you initiate the movement, so by the time you reach the top of the move you will have slowed down and the weight on the straps will have become light (but they shouldn't be slack).
● As you lower the arms to the start position, go slower than on the concentric phase rather than simply letting gravity take over.

tricks of the trade

This is an odd tip, but it works: look at the 'down' arm when you do the fly. This will make you retract the shoulder ever so slightly more than without the look.

exercise 25 single leg squat

● stability ● strength   **strap length: medium**

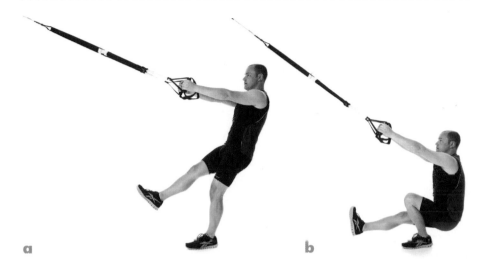

a   b

'Pistol squats' is the slightly more scary name this exercise gets given and is usually performed without weights and as deeply as possible. Getting down is easy but once you go past 90 degrees at the knee it becomes tough. However, the suspension system will make it achievable yet still very productive.

● Lean back until you are between 70 and 45 degrees V/F angle. Point the toe of one foot and lift it from the floor so that your leg is straight.
● Using just the supporting leg (avoid pulling on the straps), squat down until you reach at least a 90-degree angle at the knees.
● As you squat the handles and straps will travel up and down parallel to the depth of your squat.

tricks of the trade

If you can't get down to 90 degrees at the knee the first time you do this move, you are not alone. This is partly to do with confidence but it is also a learning curve – so start small and work up to full range if necessary.

exercise 26 t fly

● **stability** ● **strength**   **strap length: medium**

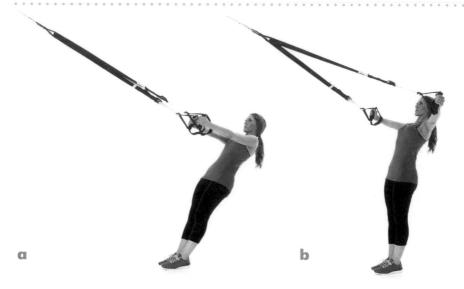

a   b

If I were in the room doing this move with you, I would make sure that you keep your arms below shoulder height and puff your chest out at the front of the movement while squeezing your shoulder blades together. I'm not there, but that's what I want you to do – and while you are at it, keep your arms straight.

● Start in a 45 degree V/F angle with your arms straight. The only obvious joints that should move are the shoulders.
● Engage the muscles in your upper back and shoulders by raising your arms wide. To ensure that your arms are in the correct position, keep your thumbs pointing upwards rather than behind you.
● When your torso is just off vertical and hands are at shoulder height, pause and slowly fold your body forwards back into the start position.

tricks of the trade
Have your thumbs pointing to the sky; this will encourage you to keep your shoulder retracted and depressed (not hunched).

exercise 27 side lunge and tap behind

• stability • strength   **strap length: medium**

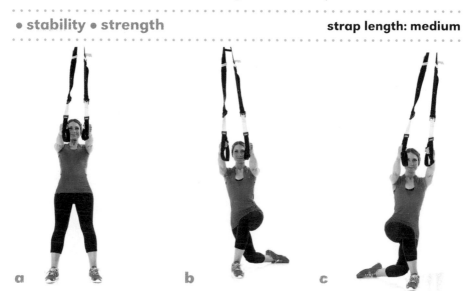

a   b   c

This move looks very dramatic if you drop down low and stretch the unloaded leg out behind you, but the plan is that you build up to that version. The suspension system actually makes this move possible because without it you would have to lean forward over the front leg rather than sitting back on to your heel.

- Most of the work is done with the front leg rather than the leg that steps back, so keep focused on the front leg.
- Begin at less than a 45 degree V/F angle. Step back, crossing the unloaded leg behind you and tap the floor with the unloaded foot.
- Keep the straps long and tight, then repeat on the other leg.

tricks of the trade

It's very tempting to pull with your arms. To overcome this instinct, let the straps go slack between each repetition (I know this breaks the no slack rule, but in this case it will improve the outcomes).

exercise 28 plank on hands

● **stability** ● **strength**   **strap length: long**

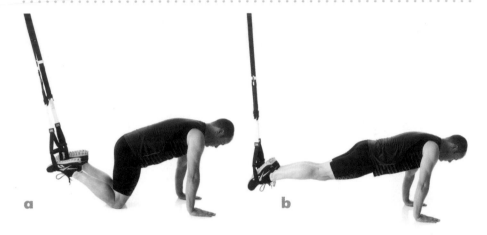

a   b

Suspended press-ups are tough: this move will help prepare you for that ultimate stage of your training. Two things happen when you add a suspension system to the plank: firstly the movement in the straps adds a challenge; and secondly the feet are raised above ground level, making it additionally challenging. Once you have tried this I doubt you will ever do a 'regular' plank again.

● Hook your feet over the foot straps, lie on your front and shuffle away from the anchor. Keep your feet slightly apart.
● Push up into the start position; your shoulders now stay at the same height throughout the exercise (there is a straight line through your shoulder, hip, knee and ankle).
● Lower your hips, thighs and abs to the floor and then lift up immediately.
● Pause in the raised position for 2–3 seconds then slowly return to the floor and repeat.

tricks of the trade
Position your hands directly under your shoulder joint so that your arms are vertical. Any angle other than 90 degrees increases the challenge.

exercise 29 supported hip hinge, 't stand'

• stability • strength   **strap length: medium**

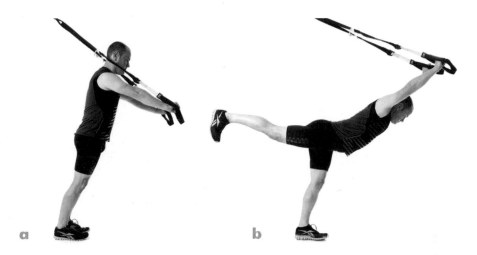

a   b

This move contains similar characteristics to some of our dynamic warm-up moves except now we add resistance to the challenge. The aim is to use your full range of shoulder mobility and hamstring flexibility and strength while balancing on one foot – sounds fun, doesn't it?

- Standing with your arms relaxed but with the straps tight, bow forwards at the waist. As you bend, simultaneously raise your arms in front of you (as if you are diving into a swimming pool).
- As soon as you start to bow, lift one leg. Keep it straight and keep lifting until it is parallel with the floor.
- When you reach your maximum range of motion, slowly reverse the movement and repeat, lifting the opposite leg.

tricks of the trade

If this move were a food, it would be classed as a 'super food'. I hardly ever see it being done in gyms, but I have included a version of it in not just this book but also in the dumbbell and kettlebell editions. It's that good!

exercise 30 triceps press, leg extension

● stability ● strength   **strap length: short**

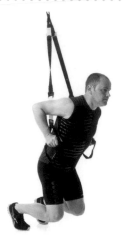
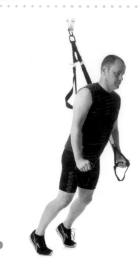

a   b

There is an extremely difficult exercise called a 'muscle-up' that is performed on Olympic rings, which requires you to pull your entire body from below the rings (pull-up position) to above them (dips position) in one swing. Our move here is nowhere near as hard but could be considered good preparation for the real deal.

● Have the straps close to your body rather than outside your forearms.
● Load the handles by taking as much weight off your feet as you can.
● Bend your elbows and legs at the same time. You need to minimise the input from your legs as this is predominantly an upper body exercise.
● When you reach 90 degrees at the elbow, push back to the top (again minimising the use of your legs).

tricks of the trade
Don't just bow forwards – you must move up and down. Look up and you should find that your head, chest and shoulders all stay in the optimum position.

exercise 31 one-handed pull

• stability • strength   **strap length: medium**

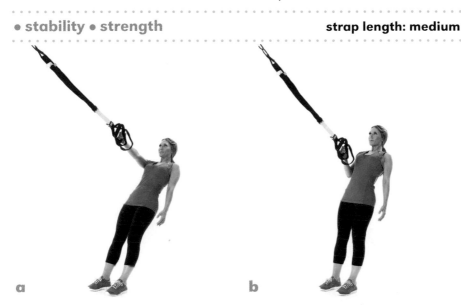

a   b

Holding just one handle rather than two introduces torsion to the list of challenges. Your feet are a fixed touch-point while the movement of the straps means that the rest of your body wants to rotate (or fall) towards its centre of gravity. With this in mind, the areas of muscle that are static (stabilising) are working just as hard as those generating movement.

- Lean backwards to a maximum of 45 degrees V/F angle while holding just one strap.
- Squat down slightly. You should feel your bodyweight on your heels and the balls of your feet.
- Keep looking up towards the anchor.
- Pull with the attached arm until your hand is almost touching your ribs, then slowly reverse the muscle action.

tricks of the trade

Your arm, abs, shoulders, upper back, glutes and hamstring are all working during this move so think of it as a 'dynamic' whole body workout rather than bicep isolation.

exercise 32 kneeling roll out

● **stability** ● **strength**   **strap length: short/medium**

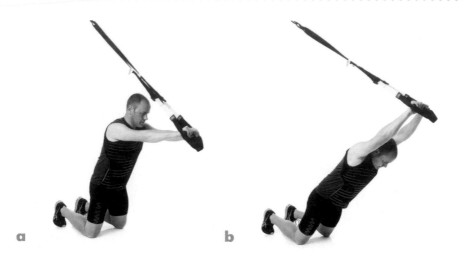

a   b

The roll out is a great exercise that I also featured in *The Total Gym Ball Workout*; on the ball you are slightly limited by the length of your arms to how much you can move, but with a suspension system you have complete freedom to move forwards, backwards and sideways making this even more effective and challenging to the shoulders and abs.

● Kneel so that the anchor is just behind you rather than straight above. Hold both handles separately and load them.
● Looking straight ahead, take the weight off your toes and very slowly dive forwards.
● When your head is level with your arms, reverse the movement.

tricks of the trade
If this move feels impossible, hold the two handles together with your thumbs to make one grip. This will give you much more control as you 'dive' forwards.

exercise 33 chest fly

● stability ● strength   **strap length: medium**

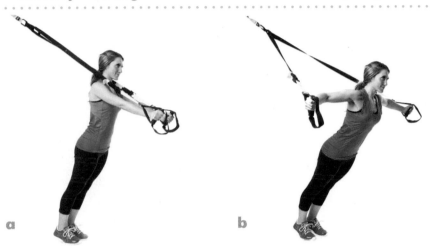

a   b

Compared to the traditional version of this move (which is performed with dumbbells) the number of muscles recruited with the suspension version is significantly more. The dumbbell purists would argue that moving through a specific range 'hits' only the chest, but frankly I'd rather hit 100+ muscles in the chest, shoulders and abs than just 10 in the chest. You do need to be a little brave in this move as you are facing the floor, so start easy and progressively work your feet back towards the anchor.

- Lean on the straps so your body is at 45 30 degrees V/F. Your arms should start and remain straight throughout the move.
- Gradually open your arms. Your body will be moving towards the floor so move slowly and keep control.
- The maximum range is reached when your hands disappear from your peripheral vision. At this point, keeping your arms straight still, drag them back together so that your body lifts back up.

tricks of the trade
If this is too tough, rather than cheating with the arms, bend your knees to shorten your overall body length – this will lighten the load on your arms.

exercise 34 foot suspended lunge

● **stability** ● **strength**   **strap length: medium**

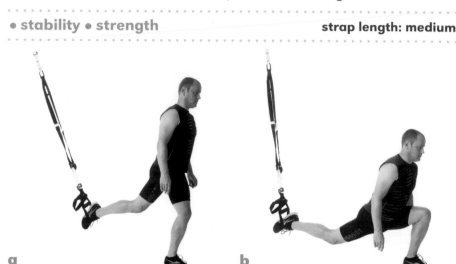

a   b

This move simply didn't exist before suspension systems became popular. After inserting your foot into the strap, you need to hop forwards until you feel your suspended leg being lifted up. Then you need to pause for just a moment before you attempt to lunge down. This is a fantastic move and like no lunge you have ever done before.

● Hook one foot into the strap and carefully hop away from the anchor point until you feel your back foot gently lifted.
● Pause until you are sure you are balanced, then squat down on the front leg. When you reach 90 degrees at the knee, stand up.
● Your suspended foot should arc back towards the anchor as you are squatting.

tricks of the trade
Make sure you press the top of your foot firmly against the strap. Not only will this help your balance, but you will feel the back leg working in a way that you have never felt before!

exercise 35 one-handed squat

• stability • strength • power   **strap length: medium**

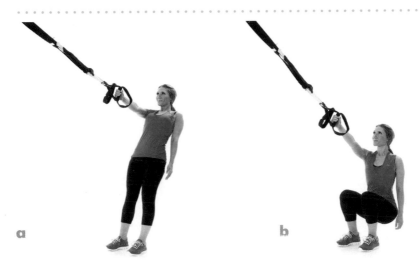

a   b

The down phase of this move is relatively unspectacular, but as you start to drive back up quickly you will experience a battle between torsion and recoil. There is a natural temptation to pull (bend) your arm, but it's best to lean back and do all the work with your legs.

- Step away from the anchor holding one handle and suspend yourself to approximately 45 degrees V/F.
- Look up at the anchor point. Your weight should be spread evenly across the front and back of your foot.
- Squat down, but don't pull on the suspension system, just let it take some of your weight.
- When you can't squat any lower, stand back up (you will most likely feel your weight shift into your heels on the way up).

tricks of the trade

When you squat down, try to touch your nearest heel with the spare hand. This will encourage your torso to slightly rotate away from the centre of gravity.

exercise 36 straight arm torso twist

• **stability** • **strength** • **power**   **strap length: medium**

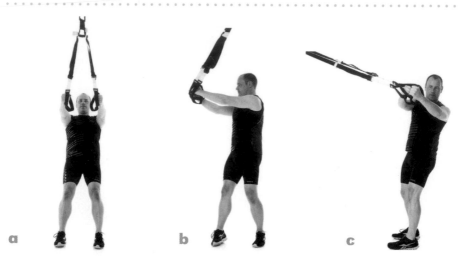

a   b   c

The essential element of this move is to keep the straps tight; as soon as they go slack, then the exercise effect is over. The fixed touch-points are your feet, but don't feel the need to keep your feet 'glued' to the floor. Let them pivot as your body moves through the arc of this torque-provoking exercise.

- Lean backwards to 70–45 degrees V/F. Both arms should be straight and at shoulder height (your chest and arms should be forming a triangle shape).
- Without changing the shape of the triangle, drive both arms to one side. Your feet stay in position, but your knees and hip both turn towards the same direction as the arms.
- Slowly return to the centre and repeat on the other side.

trickſ of the trade
Drive forwards with your glutes as you twist; if you are turning right, drive forwards with the left side, and vice versa.

exercise 37 standing roll out

● stability ● strength ● power   **strap length: short/medium**

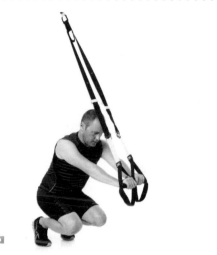

a

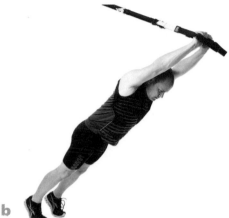

b

This move is one of those that really surprises clients (and personal trainers) when they first try it, simply because it is a big jump of intensity from the kneeling version. I classify it as a 'power' version because I want you to perform it quickly so that you are only briefly at full stretch

● Get into a low squat position with the anchor just behind you, rather than straight above. Hold both handles separately and load them.
● Looking straight ahead, push your hands firmly into the strap handles and begin to very slowly dive forwards.
● Straighten your legs until your head is level with your arms, then reverse the movement.

tricks of the trade

If this move feels daunting, hold your breath as you dive forwards. This is a natural way of stabilising the torso and, contrary to what some fitness instructors have been taught, is actually an inbuilt response to external physical demands.

exercise 38 side jumps

• stability • strength • power　　　　**strap length: medium**

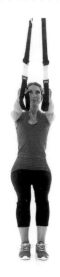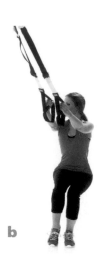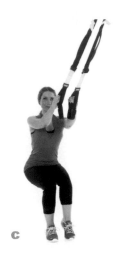

a　　　　　　　　　　b　　　　　　　　　　c

While all suspension exercises have the potential to invoke an increase in your heart rate, this move makes it unavoidable. Keep the straps tight at all times by really leaning back on them. I always relate this move to when I water ski; the temptation is to pull yourself forward when in fact you have to lean back and enjoy the ride.

- Lean back until your body is at 70–45 degrees V/F.
- Take a large step sideways, then jump back in the other direction. Bend your knees on landing to soften the impact but also increase the intensity.
- Each jump right then left counts as one repetition.

tricks of the trade

This is very much a wide jump rather than a high one so 'sit down' slightly before you push sideways and jump.

exercise 39 squat jumps

● **stability** ● **strength** ● **power**   **strap length: medium**

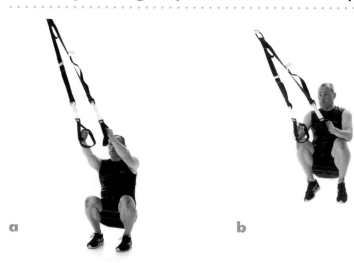

a   b

There is absolutely no hiding from the intensity of this excellent exercise. You need to lean back and let the straps take your weight – while this move isn't a true plyometric move, if you transition from the down to the up phase briskly, you should feel a definite sense of rebound as you change direction.

● Step away from the anchor until the straps are tight and your arms are at shoulder height.
● Look up at the anchor point. Your weight should be spread evenly across the front and back of your foot.
● Squat down. Don't pull on the suspension system, just let it take some of your weight. When you can't squat any lower, push back up very quickly into a jump. Due to the quick transition from down to up, the straps may go slack – this is acceptable as long as they tighten again during the next squat.

> ## **tricks of the trade**
> This really works – when you jump, rather than thinking about getting your feet off the ground, drive up with your thighs and imagine that you are leaving your feet on the floor. This way you will get a strong, more direct jump.

exercise 40 suspended abduction and adduction

• stability • strength • power   **strap length: medium**

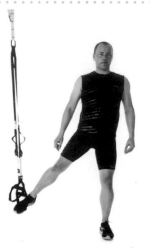
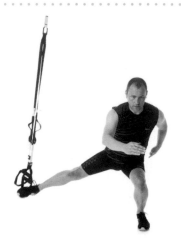

a   b

In case you are confused and thinking how can this be both abduction and adduction, the answer is when the suspended leg abducts the supporting leg adducts, and vice versa. The plan is to perform this move quickly but adhere to my mantra of 'learn it, then work it' – the amount of swing you achieve needs to be gradually increased, but only once you have learnt how to reach the high levels of inherent stability required.

- Hook one foot into the strap and carefully hop away from the anchor.
- Keep your suspended foot in plantar flexion (toes pointing down) and spread your weight between the floor and the strap.
- Let the suspended leg glide back towards the anchor and past it on the opposite V/F. You will need to bend the standing leg, however, this 'squat' is secondary to the suspended leg's gliding action.

tricks of the trade

A very simple tip but I feel the need to give you permission to do it if necessary. If you are struggling with balance on this, simply hold the strap with your nearest hand until you feel ready to let go.

exercise 41 single leg power up

• stability • strength • power　　　　　**strap length: medium**

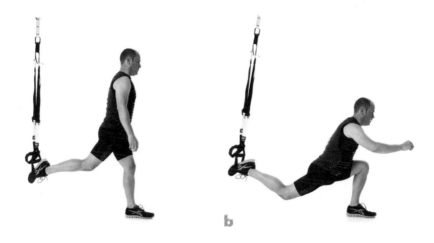

a　　　　　　　　　　　　　　　　　　b

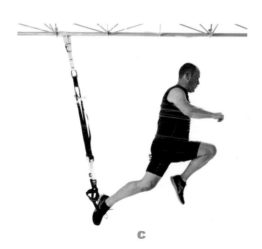

c

This is the big brother of the suspended lunge (exercise 34). This move has the potential to leave your legs quivering after just a few repetitions but it is worth it for the dynamic benefits you can achieve. Start with just a low jump then get higher as you gain confidence (note that using your arms to create momentum is not cheating).

- Hook one foot into the strap and carefully hop away from the anchor point until you feel your foot gently lifted.
- Pause until you are sure you are balanced, then squat down on the front leg.
- When you reach a maximum of 90 degrees at the knee, drive up with that leg very quickly and jump in the air.

tricks of the trade

This move is tough so you don't need to jump very high to achieve the full benefits.

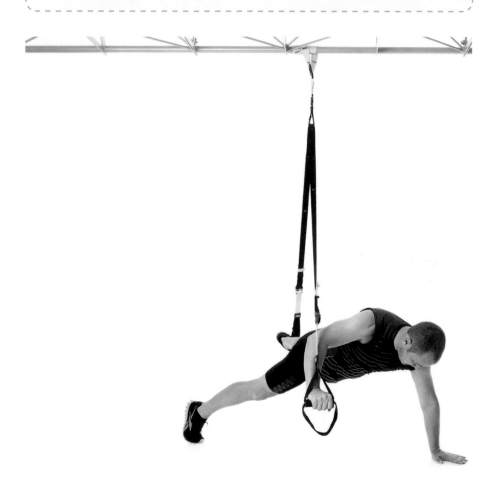

exercise 42 run ups

● **stability ● strength ● power**   **strap length: medium**

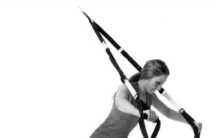

a   b

The feeling you get from this move reminds me of my track training days when we dragged a car tyre (or person) behind us as we sprinted up the track. If you fix your arms below shoulder height, the move is then pure power and cardio. Raise the touch point above your shoulders and your abs will be significantly engaged.

● You only need to lean forwards to 70 degrees V/F with your arms extended in front of you.
● From the 'ready position' (heels up, standing on the balls of your feet), start to run on the spot.
● As you build up speed make sure that you keep the straps tight.

tricks of the trade

As you get faster and faster, I notice with many clients the movement gets smaller and smaller so, as much as I hate to say it, 'get those knees up'.

exercise 43 suspended squat thrust

• stability • strength • power   **strap length: long**

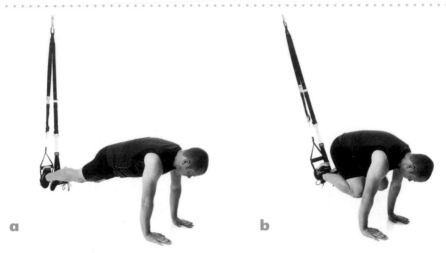

a   b

Each time you move your hands just slightly further from the anchor point you will feel this challenge increase; however, you do need to avoid having the straps completely vertical as you'll find your toes drag on the floor. Keep your hands wider than your shoulders to help your balance and lift your hips to at least the same height as your shoulders.

- Hook your feet over the foot straps, lie on your front and shuffle away from the anchor.
- Push up into the start position. Your shoulders now stay at the same height throughout the move (there is a straight line through your shoulder, hip, knee and ankle).
- Rather than shift your bodyweight onto your hands, keep some force pushing down into the foot loops.
- Now, quickly bring both knees towards your chest, then quickly drive them back to the start position.

tricks of the trade
Your hips will lift up as you build up speed. This isn't bad but will reduce the amount of abdominal activity so stay as 'flat' as possible.

exercise 44 suspended squat thrust and swing

● **stability** ● **strength** ● **power**   **strap length: long**

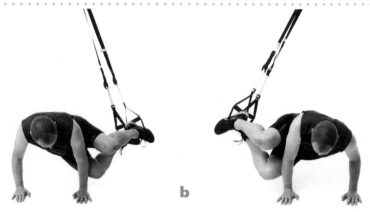

a   b

This move looks pretty spectacular but personally I think there are harder moves that look more innocent. Saying that though, this is a great move for muscle recruitment and power development. The further you place your hands from the anchor the tougher it becomes, but if you venture too far away, the tension in the straps will stop you from being able to bring your knees towards your chest at all.

● Hook your feet over the foot straps, lie on your front, and shuffle away from the anchor.
● Push up into the start position. Your shoulders now stay at the same height throughout the exercise (there is a straight line through your shoulder, hip, knee and ankle).
● Rather than shift weight onto your hands, keep some force pushing down into the foot loops.
● Now, quickly swing both legs towards one arm (ultimately aim for the outside of the elbow). Then, without returning to the start position, swing the legs to the other side.

tricks of the trade
This move is as much about controlling the swing as it is about generating it so I'd rather see a tight, controlled move than legs swaying all over the place.

exercise 45 suspended pike

• **stability** • **strength** • **power**   **strap length: long**

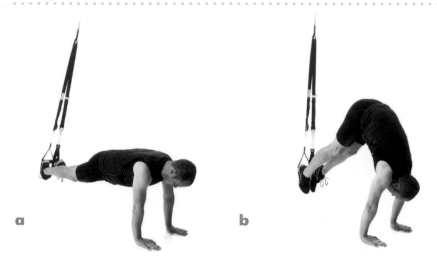

a   b

Your ability to do this move will only be as good as your technique on the down dog stretch so it's a good idea to perform a few reps of that before going for the pike. I've listed this move in the power section because a) I want it performed fast; and b) unless you have developed the skill and strength on the less challenging moves, it's a lot to ask of you.

● Hook both feet into the straps, shuffle away from the anchor and lift up into the suspended plank position.
● While keeping your legs straight, raise your hips as high as you can.
● Then, with control, slowly lower them back into the plank position.

tricks of the trade
You will instinctively want to bend your knees in this move. To overcome that temptation you need to press harder with your hands and arms.

exercise 46 alternate leg hamstring curl

• stability • strength • power   **strap length: long**

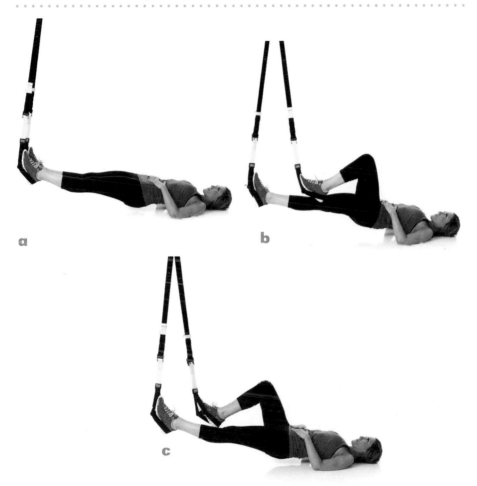

Being suspended directly below the anchor point tends to make your legs swing like a pendulum side to side (while not a bad thing it's not adding anything to the move), so shuffle your body away from the anchor. You must get into a high bridge position to really get the most out of this move and go as fast as you can without losing the quality of movement.

● Place your feet in the foot straps while directly under the anchor point, then shuffle your body backwards.

- Lift your hips up. Your touch-points are the heels and shoulders, but if you find yourself swinging excessively from side to side, then keep your elbows touching the ground as shown – again, avoid pressing your head hard against the floor.
- Bend one leg until your heels are as close to your glutes as possible, then lengthen that leg and repeat with the other leg.

> ### tricks of the trade
>
> As you build up speed, the crossover of the two feet will creep further from the anchor point and the range of movement has a bad habit of reducing – so a rep only counts if you straighten the leg every time!

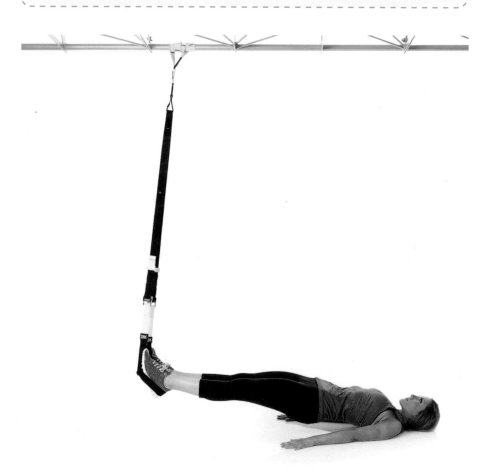

exercise 47 single leg side lunge with no touch

• stability • strength • power　　　　**strap length: medium**

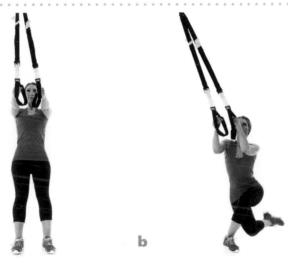

a　　　　　　　　　　　　　　　b

This is the progression of the side lunge and tap behind move (exercise 27). At any time you only have three touch-points so the challenge is increased significantly. While the leg extending behind and to the side looks impressive, our focus is the depth of the single leg lunge. You do need a slight bend in your elbows to enable the rotation to occur.

- Most of the work is done with the front leg rather than the leg that steps back, so keep focused on the front leg.
- Begin at less than a 45 degree V/F angle. Step back crossing the unloaded leg stretched behind you, but don't touch the floor.
- Keep the straps long and tight. To change to the other leg, you need to jump and swap feet – it's very tempting to pull with your arms but resist this as much as possible.

tricks of the trade

It's cool to get some rotation into this move. To maximise this, let one handle drop lower than the other – if you are stood on your left foot, it will be the left hand).

exercise 48 balance lunge and knee drive

• **stability** • **strength** • **power**   **strap length: medium**

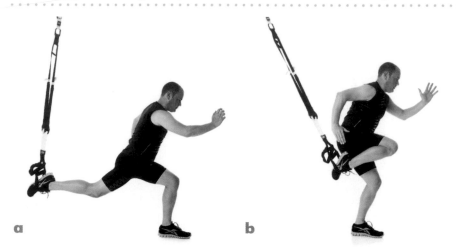

a   b

When you keep the straps tight, the handles are always moving through a curve. On this move you want the curve to be as big as possible; to achieve this you need to maintain downward pressure on the handle throughout the knee drive phase of the move (that's forwards and backwards).

- Hook one foot into the strap and carefully hop away from the anchor point until you start to feel your foot being lifted.
- Pause until you are sure you are balanced, then squat down a little on the front leg. Your suspended foot needs to maintain pressure on the suspension system at all times.
- Now, drive the suspended leg in front of you. Pumping your arms in time with the leg action will add to the intensity and help you balance.

tricks of the trade
Really drive hard with your arms to amplify the leg action – my running coach used to shout at me, 'You've got four legs, two on your butt and two on your shoulders!'

exercise 49 suspended press-up

● **stability** ● **strength** ● **power**   **strap length: long**

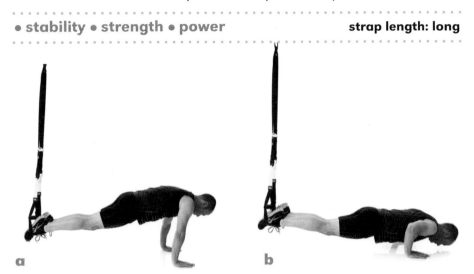

a   b

I've set the strap length as 'long' to begin with, however, as you improve note that raising them will progressively and significantly increase the challenge. You can keep raising them up to the point that you are performing a supported handstand press-up – however, most people perform that version poorly because it is an 'all or nothing' move.

● Hook both feet into the straps, shuffle away from the anchor and lift up into the suspended plank position. Keep your feet slightly apart.
● Bend your elbows to lower your chest towards the floor. (Because your feet are raised, you will find that you won't achieve the same parallel to the floor position that you do with a regular press-up – this is fine).
● When you reach the lowest point, push back up to the start position.

tricks of the trade

Unlike on a regular press-up where your lower body is relaxed when suspended, you need to activate more of your leg muscles to create stability, so 'squeeze' with your quads and shin muscles throughout both the up and down phase.

103

exercise 50 one-handed squat and pull

● **stability** ● **strength** ● **power**   **strap length: medium**

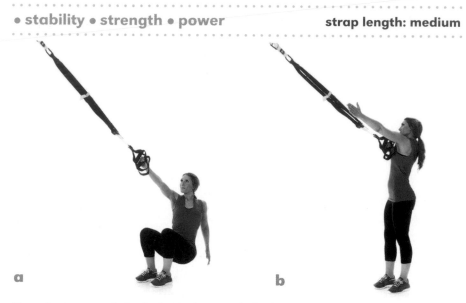

a   b

There isn't a muscle in the body that can hide during this exercise. The intensity is infinitely adjustable by stepping closer to the anchor or reaching further behind yourself on the squat section.

● Holding one handle, step away from the anchor and suspend yourself to approximately 45 degrees V/F.
● Look up at the anchor point. Your weight should be spread evenly across the front and back of your foot.
● Squat down, but don't pull on the suspension system – just let it take some of your weight.
● When you can't squat any lower, stand back up and simultaneously pull with the arm holding the handle. With the free hand reach up towards the anchor point.

tricks of the trade
If you think you might be able to perform this as a single-legged version, start by splitting your feet then predominately load just the front leg.

exercise 51 pike press-up

• stability • strength • power   **strap length: long**

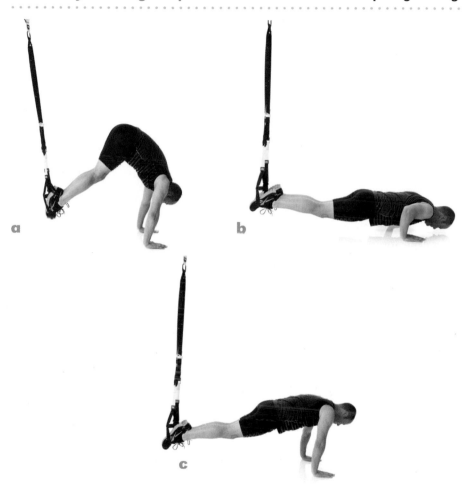

The pike section will challenge your arms, chest, shoulders and abdominals, then the press-up goes after the same muscles but prioritises them differently – however you think about this, it is a tough exercise but also highly rewarding.

- Hook both feet into the straps, shuffle away from the anchor and lift up into the suspended plank position.
- Keeping your legs straight, raise your hips as high as you can; then, with control, slowly lower them back into the plank position.

105

- As soon as your body is parallel to the floor, bend your elbows and lower down and then up for the press-up section of this move.

> ### tricks of the trade
>
> This move is best performed without any 'punctuation'. By that I mean each phase should just blend together rather than being split up by pauses. As soon as you start to 'unfold' the pike, start to lower down into the press-up.

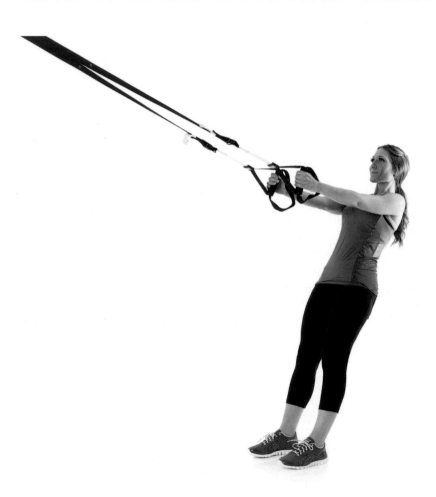

exercise 52 seated pull-up

● stability ● strength ● power   **strap length: short**

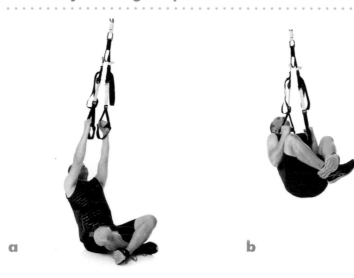

a   b

This is the 'easy' version of this exercise; the tough method is to do the same technique with the upper body but with your legs extended out straight in front of you. Make sure that you control the muscle action in both directions – don't just get to the top then drop to the floor with a thud.

● Sit cross-legged under the anchor point. Lean back and look up towards the anchor.
● Squeeze your knees and ankles together so that they stay 'bonded' throughout the lift.
● Pull your body off the floor until your chest is touching the handles, then slowly, with good control, lower back down.

tricks of the trade

With this move, the rule is the faster the better. Going slow is very artificial and something we tend to only do on mechanical gym equipment – so for this to be a 'transferable skill', hit it fast and hard.

crazy stuff that I won't ask you to do

 exercise 53 2 x suspended system squats

strap length: long

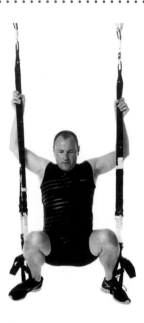

 tricks of the trade

Do the pike press-up (exercise 51, page 105) instead. I know it looks very different, but, in terms of muscle recruitment, this is similar and also better because the hands are loaded rather than gripping the vertical axis.

exercise 54 anything that involves a handstand

strap length: medium

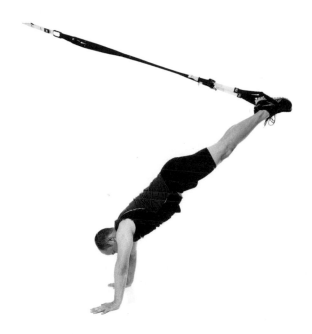

tricks of the trade

I will make an exception here if you are performing the handstand on a very soft surface like sand. However, I have seen so many people headbutt the floor while doing this, so I think it's rather risky. My preferred option is to do the standing roll out (exercise 37, page 89) instead.

exercise 55 suspended side plank on
one elbow

strap length: medium

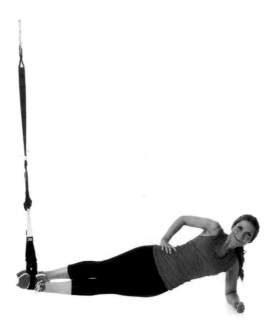

 ### tricks of the trade

This is a common exercise; however, I find that even with a mat the pressure on the supporting elbow is too uncomfortable to be good. As an alternative do the straight arm torso twist (exercise 36, page 88) instead.

exercise 56 suspended one-hand
one-foot press-up

strap length: long

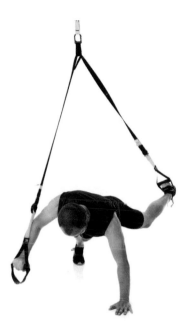

 tricks of the trade

I'm not being stubborn here but I find it really hard to think how this move provides 'transferable' skills. It's very hard and not particularly dangerous – but there is a chance you will just end up flat on the floor! Do the suspended squat thrust and swing (exercise 44, page 97) instead.

exercise 57 feet on the wall press ups

strap length: medium

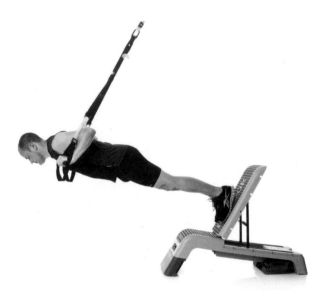

 ### tricks of the trade

As soon as you put your feet up the wall, you lose some of the vertical down force so the increased challenge that you would experience is all about gripping the wall rather than the effects of being suspended. Do the suspended press-up (exercise 49, page 103) instead.

exercise 58 feet on the wall row

strap length: medium

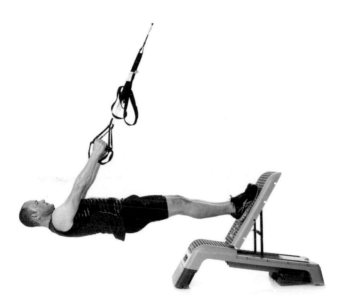

 tricks of the trade

Do the seated pull-up (exercise 52, page 107) instead. As before, having the feet against the wall doesn't add anything productive to this move, so unless you want footprints up the wall, don't do it. The alternative is much better.

3 training with a suspension system

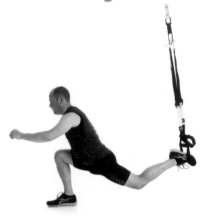

how to use the suspension training sessions

. . . .

As people become more experienced in training with suspension systems there is a temptation to forego a formal training plan and work through a session training body parts randomly. This can be effective, but human nature dictates that, given the opportunity, we often end up focusing on the parts we like to work rather than the parts we need to work.

The training sessions in this section follow the S.A.F.E. philosophy of progression, and are divided into the three basic facets of this system: stability, strength and power. They are sequenced in such a way that if you were an absolute beginner when you started, you should have at least 18 months of progressive exercise experience before you perform the hardest session. So, a novice would first attempt the 15-minute stability session followed, when ready, by the 30-minute and then 45-minute sessions. This process could take three to six months. When the stability sessions have been mastered and no longer present a significant challenge, the 15-minute strength session can be attempted, followed, when ready, by the 30- and 45-minute sessions; again, this process could take three to six months. Having developed stability and strength over this length of time the body will be well-prepared to progress to the power sessions, which follow the same logical progressions. Note: The timings are approximate and include a short warm-up and stretching at the end of the session.

The reality is, of course, that many people are not complete beginners, so Table 3 gives you an idea of where to start depending upon your experience and physical ability.

Table 3 Assessing which training session to begin with	
Stage	**Where to start**
You have not used a suspension system on a regular basis	If so, that makes you a novice – start with the stability sessions before progressing to strength then power
You have been using a suspension system for 6–18 months and can do a perfect overhead squat	If so, that makes you experienced – you might benefit from doing the stability sessions, but you can start with the strength sessions before progressing to the power sessions
You have been using a suspension system for 18 months or more and can do a perfect overhead squat	If so, you might benefit from doing the stability and strength sessions, but you can start with the power sessions

the warm-up

Before you start any of the workouts, you need to do a warm-up. This can vary depending upon where you are – in a gym you might choose to use the cardio equipment (treadmill, rower, cross-trainer) to get ready. This is fine; however, I find the most effective warm-up is one that specifically mimics the work that is about to be done, so I like to prepare by going through movements that feature in the actual workout, e.g. full range versions of light squats, rotation and shoulder movements, along with some temperature-raising activities such as jogging on the spot.

post-workout stretch

In the world of fitness we habitually stretch at the end of our workout sessions when the muscles are still warm. However, muscles will also be fatigued and therefore not particularly receptive to being stretched. The reality is that most people just want to get out of the door when they have finished the work section, and they view stretching as something that delays their shower, so I like to do the essential stretches just after the workout, then make time when less fatigued to do some more quality, focused flexibility work.

The effects of stretching are cumulative so don't expect miracles the first time, or if you really struggle to make time for them, remember that the reason for warming up and stretching at the end of every session is to reduce the risk of injury. So, make a habit of incorporating stretching into your workout, or risk paying for the privilege of a physiotherapist telling you the same thing in the future.

You should complete the following essential stretches at the end of every exercise session (see below). Hold each of the stretches for at least 20 seconds and try to relax and enjoy them.

stretch 1 Suspended hip stretch

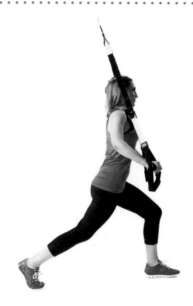

stretch 2 Supported inner thigh

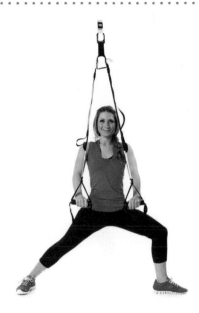

stretch 3 Suspended 'C' stretch

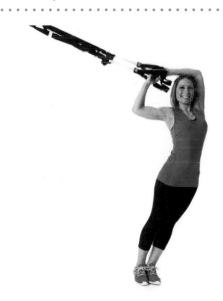

stretch 4 Supported back extension

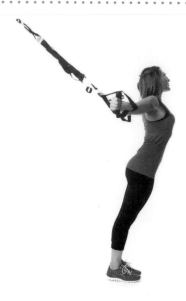

stretch 5 Supported down dog

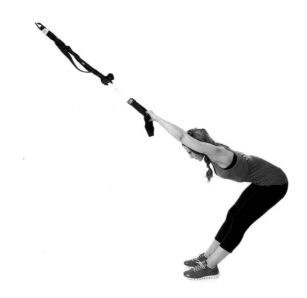

the workouts

the dynamic warm-up

The dynamic warm-up precedes all of the suspension system training workout sessions. Perform each of the warm-up moves in sequence for at least 30-60 seconds per move or for as long as it takes your muscles and joints to feel ready for action (see pages 52–56).

1 Upper back dynamic stretch
2 Dynamic chest stretch
3 Low back dynamic stretch
4 Torso shoulder rotation
5 Little jumps

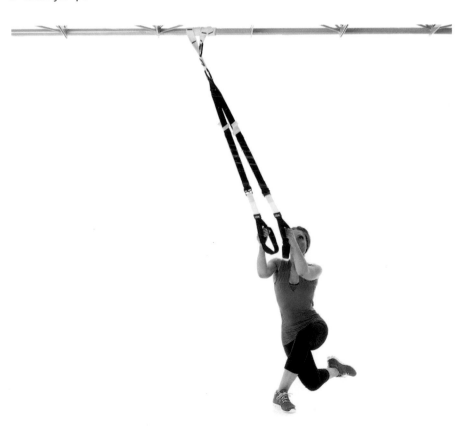

stability workout sessions

15-minute stability (2 circuits)	
Order in which to do moves	**Technique**
exercise 6 row (page 57) 15 reps	
exercise 11 side lunge (page 62) 15 reps	
exercise 7 chest press (page 58) 15 reps	
exercise 19 squat, back to anchor (page 70) 15 reps	
exercise 20 hip dip (page 71) 15 reps	
exercise 16 bridge (page 67) 15 reps	

exercise 13 prone plank on elbows (page 64) 10 reps	
exercise 14 supine plank (page 65) 10 reps	

20-minute stability (2 circuits)

Order in which to do moves	Technique
exercise 10 bicep curl (page 61) 15 reps	
exercise 9 back extension (page 60) 15 reps	
exercise 8 squat (page 59) 15 reps	
exercise 12 triceps press (page 63) 15 reps	

exercise 6 row (page 57) 15 reps	
exercise 20 hip dip (page 71) 15 reps	
exercise 18 lunge step back (page 69) 15 reps	
exercise 17 hamstring curl (page 68) 15 reps	
exercise 13 prone plank on elbows (page 64) 10 reps	
exercise 16 suspended bridge (page 67) 15 reps	

30-minute stability (2 circuits)	
Order in which to do moves	**Technique**
exercise 6 row (page 57) 15 reps	
exercise 10 bicep curl (page 61) 15 reps	
exercise 7 chest press (page 58) 15 reps	
exercise 20 hip dip (page 71) 15 reps	
exercise 12 triceps press (page 63) 15 reps	
exercise 9 back extension (page 60) 15 reps	

exercise 17 hamstring curl (page 68) 15 reps	
exercise 16 suspended bridge (page 67) 15 reps	
exercise 11 side lunge (page 62) 10 reps	
exercise 14 supine plank (page 65) 10 reps	
exercise 15 balance lunge (page 66) 15 reps	
exercise 19 squat, back to anchor (page 70) 15 reps	

strength workout sessions

15-minute strength (2 circuits)	
Order in which to do moves	**Technique**
exercise 21 y fly (page 73) 15 reps	
exercise 27 side lunge and tap behind (page 79) 15 reps	
exercise 26 t fly (page 78) 15 reps	
exercise 25 single leg squat (page 77) 15 reps	
exercise 29 supported hip hinge, 't stand' (page 81) 15 reps	
exercise 22 overhead squat, facing anchor (page 74) 15 reps	

exercise 31 one-handed pull (page 83) 15 reps	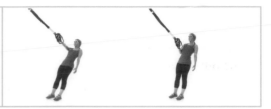

20-minute strength (2 circuits)	
Order in which to do moves	**Technique**
exercise 24 x fly (page 76) 15 reps	
exercise 23 overhead squat, back to anchor (page 75) 15 reps	
exercise 33 chest fly (page 85) 15 reps	
exercise 34 foot suspended lunge (page 86) 15 reps	
exercise 28 plank on hands (page 80) 10 reps	

exercise 17 hamstring curl (page 68) 15 reps	
exercise 32 kneeling roll out (page 84) 10 reps	
exercise 30 tricep press, leg extension (page 82) 15 reps	
exercise 31 one-handed pull (page 83) 15 reps	
exercise 20 hip dip (page 71) 15 reps	

30-minute strength (2 circuits)	
Order in which to do moves	**Technique**
exercise 21 y fly (page 73) 15 reps	
exercise 31 one-handed pull (page 83) 15 reps	
exercise 27 side lunge and tap behind (page 79) 15 reps	
exercise 34 foot suspended lunge (page 86) 15 reps	
exercise 33 chest fly (page 85) 10 reps	
exercise 29 supported hip hinge, 't stand' (page 81) 15 reps	

exercise 32 kneeling roll out (page 84) 10 reps	
exercise 22 overhead squat, facing anchor (page 74) 15 reps	
exercise 25 single leg squat (page 77) 15 reps	
exercise 20 hip dip (page 71) 15 reps	
exercise 28 plank on hands (page 80) 10 reps	

power workout sessions

15-minutes power (2 circuits: 1st circuit ● 10 reps; 2nd circuit ● 15 reps)	
Order in which to do moves	**Technique**
exercise 35 one-handed squat (page 87)	
exercise 38 side jumps (page 90)	
exercise 36 straight arm torso twist (page 88)	
exercise 42 run ups (page 95)	
exercise 40 suspended abduction and adduction (page 92)	
exercise 49 suspended press-up (page 103)	

exercise 46 alternate leg hamstring curl (page 99)	
exercise 43 suspended squat thrust (page 96)	

20-minutes power (2 circuits: 1st circuit ● 10 reps; 2nd circuit ● 15 reps)	
Order in which to do moves	**Technique**
exercise 50 one-handed squat and pull (page 104)	
exercise 37 standing roll out (page 89)	
exercise 39 squat jumps (page 91)	
exercise 45 suspended pike (page 98)	

exercise 47 single leg side lunge with no touch (page 101)	
exercise 21 y fly (page 73)	
exercise 48 balance lunge and knee drive (page 102)	
exercise 22 overhead squat, facing anchor (page 74)	
exercise 46 alternate leg hamstring curl (page 99)	
exercise 51 pike press-up (page 105)	

30-minutes power (2 circuits: 1st circuit ● 10 reps; 2nd circuit ● 15 reps)	
Order in which to do moves	**Technique**
exercise 50 one-handed squat and pull (page 104)	
exercise 26 t fly (page 78)	
exercise 41 single leg power up (page 93)	
exercise 40 suspended abduction and adduction (page 92)	
exercise 44 suspended squat thrust and swing (page 97)	
exercise 46 alternate leg hamstring curl (page 99)	

exercise 37 standing roll out (page 89)	
exercise 36 straight arm torso twist (page 88)	
exercise 39 squat jumps (page 91)	
exercise 42 run ups (page 95)	
exercise 51 pike press-up (page 105)	
exercise 52 seated pull-up (page 107)	

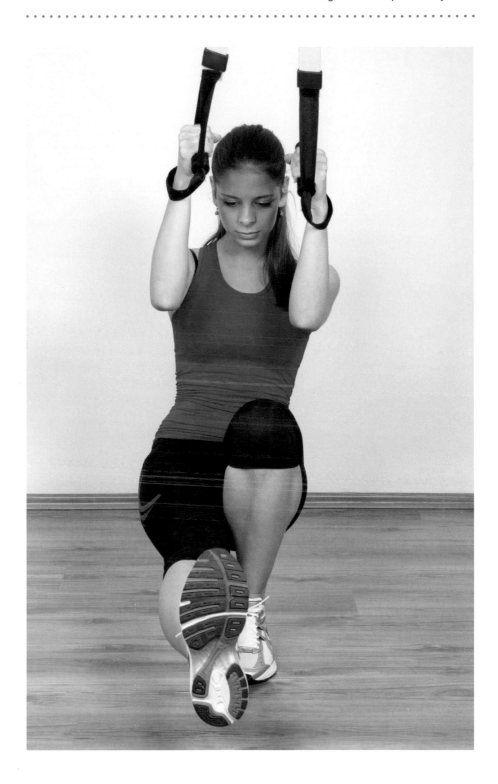

and finally...

Suspension Training Systems® have, in a very short time, gone from being something that few people had ever tried to being one of the most popular items of fitness equipment for home and gymnasiums. The possibilities are endless and, no matter what your goals, a suspension system can play a significant part in helping you to achieve them.

Whether you are a personal trainer, sportsperson or fitness enthusiast, I hope you are now fully equipped to get the most out of the valuable time you spend doing exercise with your chosen system, whether it is a simple set of gymnastic rings or one of the purpose-made adjustable commercial systems. All I ask is that you use all the information I have given in this book and make it part of an integrated health- and fitness-driven lifestyle. My many thousands of hours spent in gymnasiums, health clubs, sports fields and with personal training clients has taught me that, given the chance, people like to do the things they are already good at. So before you reach your maximum potential training with a suspension system, the smart ones among you will be looking to introduce new challenges with different equipment like dumbbells, barbells, medicine balls or suspension systems, as well as new challenges for cardiovascular fitness and flexibility.

As a personal trainer I know that I have a greater-than-average interest in the human body and the effects of exercise, partly because it is my passion and partly because it is my job. I also recognise that in the busy world we live in, expecting the same level of interest and dedication from clients towards health and exercise is unrealistic, so for me the best personal trainers are those who help clients to integrate exercise into everyday life rather than allow it to dominate.

The body is an amazing thing and responds to exercise by adapting and improving the way that it functions. Exercise is not all about pain, challenges and hard work; rather it is about making sure that in the long term your life includes the elements that have the greatest effect. I strongly believe that every minute you invest in exercise pays you back with interest, and that it's all about finding the right balance – which, in a book about exercising with one of the best products available for improving balance, is a good thought to end on.

Finding that balance is different for all of us, but you can't go far wrong if you train for stability, strength and maybe power. Walk and run, eat healthily and drink water. Find time to relax and stretch, but above all remember: if you ever find yourself lacking in motivation, the best advice I can give anybody wanting to feel healthier is that if you're moving, you're improving.

fitness glossary

As a person interested in health and fitness there is no need to sound like you have swallowed a textbook for breakfast. Yes, you need to understand how things work, but I feel there is more skill in being able to explain complicated subjects in simple language rather than simply memorising a textbook. The following glossary sets out to explain the key words and phrases that, for a person interested in the body, are useful to know and that will help you get the most out of this book, especially the training section.

Abdominals The name given to the group of muscles that make up the front of the torso, also known as the abs.

Abduction The opposite of **adduction**. The term the medical profession uses to describe any movement of a limb away from the midline of the body. So, if you raise your arm up to the side, that would be described as 'abduction of the shoulder'.

Acceleration The opposite of **deceleration**. The speed at which a movement increases from start to finish. When using weights, accelerating the weight instead of moving it at a constant speed really adds to the challenge.

Adduction The opposite of **abduction**. The term the medical profession uses to describe any movement of a limb across the midline of the body. So, if you cross your legs, that would be 'adduction of the hip'.

Aerobic The opposite of **anaerobic**. The word invented in 1968 by Dr Kenneth Cooper to describe the process in our body when we are working 'with oxygen'. While the term is now associated with the dance-based exercise to music (ETM), the original aerobic exercises that Cooper measured were cross-country running, skiing, swimming, running, cycling and walking. Generally most people consider activity up to 80 per cent of **maximum heart rate (MHR)** to be aerobic and beyond that to be anaerobic.

Age The effects of exercise change throughout life. With strength training in particular age will influence the outcome. As you reach approximately the age of 40, maintaining and developing lean muscle mass becomes harder and, in fact, the body starts to lose lean mass as a natural part of the ageing process. This can be combated somewhat with close attention to diet and exercise. At the other end of the scale a sensible approach is required when introducing very young people to training with weights.

Personally I don't like to see children participating in very heavy weight training, as it should not be pursued by boys and girls who are still growing (in terms of bone structure, rather than muscle structure). Excessive loading on prepubescent bones may have an adverse effect. There is very little conclusive research available on this subject, as it would require children to be put through tests that require them to lift very heavy weights in order to assess how much is too much. Newborn babies have over 300 bones and as we grow some bones fuse together leaving an adult with an average of 206 mature bones by age 20.

Agility Your progressive ability to move at speed and change direction while doing so.

Anaerobic The opposite of **aerobic**. High intensity bursts of cardiovascular activity generally above 80 per cent of MHR. The term literally means 'without oxygen' because when operating at this speed, the body flicks over to the fuel stored in muscles rather than mixing the fuel first with oxygen, which is what happens during aerobic activity.

Anaerobic threshold The point at which the body cannot clear lactic acid fast enough to avoid a build-up in the bloodstream. The delaying of this occurrence is a major characteristic of performance athletes. Their frequent high-intensity training increases (delays) the point at which this waste product becomes overwhelming.

Assessment I like to say that if you don't assess, you guess, so before embarking on any exercise regime you should assess your health and fitness levels in a number of areas, which can include flexibility, range of motion, strength or any of the cardiac outputs that can be measured at home or in the laboratory.

Barbell A long bar (6–7ft) with disc weights loaded onto each end. Olympic bars are competition-grade versions that rotate on bearings to enable very heavy weights to be lifted.

Biceps The muscle at the front of the upper arm. They make up about one-third of the entire diameter of the upper arm with the triceps forming the other two-thirds.

Blood pressure When the heart contracts and squirts out blood the pressure on the walls of the blood vessels is the blood pressure. It is expressed as a fraction, for example 130/80. The 130 (systolic) is the high point of the pressure being exerted on the tubes and the 80 (diastolic) is the lower amount of pressure between the main pulses.

Body Pump® A group exercise programme available in health clubs that changed the way people think about lifting weights simply by using music for timing and motivation. Rather than counting the reps, the class follows the set tunes and work around all the different muscle groups as the music tracks change.

Cardiovascular system (CV) This is the superhighway around the body. Heart, lungs and blood vessels transport and deliver the essentials of life: oxygen, energy, nutrients. Having delivered all this good stuff it then removes the rubbish by transporting away the waste products from the complex structure of muscle tissue.

Centre line An imaginary line that runs down the centre of the body from the chin to a point through the ribs, pelvis, right down to the floor.

Circuit A list of exercises can be described as a circuit. If you see '2 circuits' stated on a programme, it means you are expected to work through that list of exercises twice.

Concentric contraction The opposite of **eccentric contraction**. If this word isn't familiar to you just think 'contract', as in to get smaller/shorter.
    A concentric contraction is when a muscle shortens under tension. For example, when you lift a cup towards your mouth you produce a concentric contraction of the bicep (don't make the mistake of thinking that when you lower the cup it's a concentric contraction of the opposite muscle, i.e. the triceps – it's an eccentric movement of the bicep).

Contact points The parts of the body that are touching the bench, ball, wall or floor. The smaller the contact points, e.g. heels rather than entire foot, the greater the balance and stabilisation requirements of an exercise.

Core Ah, the core. Ask 10 trainers to describe the core and you will get 10 different answers. To me it is the obvious muscles of the abdominals, the lower back, etc., but it is also the smaller deep muscles and connective tissue that provide stability and strength to the individual. Muscles such as the glutes, hamstrings and, most importantly, the pelvic floor are often overlooked as playing a key role in the core. When I am doing a demonstration of core muscle activation, the way I sum up the core is that the majority of movements that require stability are in some way using all of the muscles that connect between the nipples and the knees.

Creatine An amino acid created naturally in your body. Every time you perform any intense exercise e.g. weight training, your body uses creatine as a source of energy. The body has the ability to store more creatine than it produces, so taking it as a supplement would allow you to train for longer at high intensity. Consuming creatine is only productive when combined with high intensity training and, therefore, is not especially relevant until you start to train for power.

Cross training An excellent approach to fitness training where you use a variety of methods to improve your fitness, rather than just one. Cross training is now used by athletes and sportspeople to reduce injury levels, as it ensures that you have a balanced amount of cardio, strength and flexibility training in a schedule.

Deceleration The opposite of **acceleration**. It is the decrease in velocity of an object. If you consider that injuries in sportspeople more often occur during the deceleration phase rather than the acceleration phase of their activity (for example, a sprinter pulling up at the end of the race, rather than when they push out of the starting blocks), you will focus particularly on this phase of all the moves in this book. The power moves especially call for you to control the 'slowing down' part of the move, which requires as much skill as it does to generate the speed in the first place.

Delayed onset muscle soreness (DOMS) This is that unpleasant muscle soreness that you get after starting a new kind of activity or when you have worked harder than normal. It was once thought that the soreness was caused by lactic acid becoming 'trapped' in the muscle after a workout, but we now realise that this is simply not the case because lactic acid doesn't hang around – it is continuously moved and metabolised. The pain is far more likely to be caused by a mass of tiny little muscle tears. It's not a cure, but some light exercise will often ease the pain because this increases the flow of blood and nutrients to the damaged muscle tissue.

Deltoid A set of three muscles that sit on top of your shoulders.

Dumbbell A weight designed to be lifted with one hand. It can be adjustable or of a fixed weight, and the range of weights available goes from a rather pointless 1kg up to a massive 50kg plus.

Dynamometer A little gadget used to measure strength by squeezing a handheld device that measures the force of your grip.

Dyna-Band® A strip of rubber used as an alternative to a dumbbell, often by physiotherapists for working muscles through specific ranges of motion where weights are either too intense or can't target the appropriate muscles. Dyna-Bands® can be held flat against the skin to give subtle muscle stimulation; for example, by wrapping a strip around the shoulders (like an Egyptian mummy), you can then work through protraction and retraction movements of the shoulder girdle.

Eccentric contraction The opposite of **concentric contraction**. The technical term for when a muscle is lengthening under tension. An easy example to remember is the lowering of a dumbbell during a bicep curl, which is described as an eccentric contraction of the bicep.

Eye line Where you are looking when performing movements. Some movement patterns are significantly altered by correct or incorrect eye line; for example, if the eye line is too high during squats, then the head is lifted and the spine will experience excessive extension.

Fascia Connective tissue that attaches muscles to muscles and enables individual muscle fibres to be bundled together. While not particularly scientific, a good way to visualise fascia is that it performs in a similar way to the skin of a sausage by keeping its contents where it should be.

Fitball (gym ball, stability ball, Swiss ball) The large balls extensively used for stability training by therapists and in gyms. They are available in sizes 55–75cm. If you are using them for weight training always remember to add your weight and the dumbbell weight together to make sure the total weight doesn't exceed the safety limit of the ball.

Flexibility The misconception is that we do flexibility to stretch the muscle fibres and make them longer, whereas, in fact, when we stretch effectively it is the individual muscle fibres that end up moving more freely against each other, creating a freer, increased range of motion.

Foam rolling This is a therapy technique that has become mainstream. You use a cylinder of foam to massage your own muscles (generally you sit or lie on the roller to exert force via your bodyweight). Interestingly, while this has a positive effect on your muscle fibres, it is the fascia that is 'stretched' most. Foam rolling is actually rather painful when you begin, but as you improve, the pain decreases. Often used by athletes as part of their warm-up.

Free weights The collective name for dumbbells and barbells. There has been a huge influx of new products entering this category so in the free weights area of a good gym you will also find kettlebells and medicine balls. In bodybuilding gyms you will often find items not designed for exercise but which are challenging to lift and use, such as heavy chains, ropes and tractor tyres.

Functional training Really all training should be functional as it is the pursuit of methods and movements that benefit you in day-to-day life. Therefore, squats are functionally beneficial for your abdominals because they work them in conjunction with other muscles, but sit-ups are not because they don't work the abdominals in a way that relates to many everyday movements.

Gait Usually associated with running and used to describe the way that a runner hits the ground either with the inside, centre or outside of their foot and, specifically, how the foot, ankle and knee joints move. However, this term also relates to how you stand and walk. Mechanical issues that exist below the knee can have a knock-on effect on other joints and muscles throughout the body. Pronation is the name given to the natural inward roll of the ankle that occurs when the heel strikes the ground and the foot flattens out. Supination refers to the opposite outward roll that occurs during the push-off phase of the walking and running movement. A mild amount of pronation and supination is both healthy and necessary to propel the body forward.

Genes Genes can influence everything from your hair colour to your predisposition to developing diseases. Clearly there is nothing you can do to influence your genes, so accept that some athletes are born great because they have the odds stacked on their side while others have to train their way to glory.

Gluteus maximus A set of muscles on your bottom, also known as the glutes.

Hamstring A big set of muscles down the back of the thigh. It plays a key role in core stability and needs to be flexible if you are to develop a good squat technique.

Heart rate (HR) Also called 'the pulse'. It is the number of times each minute that your heart contracts. An athlete's HR could be as low as 35 beats per minute (BPM) when resting but can also go up to 250BPM during activity. See also **Resting heart rate**.

Hypertrophy The growth of skeletal muscle. This is what a bodybuilder is constantly trying to achieve. The number of muscle fibres we have is fixed, so rather than 'growing' new muscles fibres hypertrophy is the process of increasing the size of the existing fibre. Building muscle is a slow and complex process that requires constant training and a detailed approach to nutrition.

Insertion All muscles are attached to bone or other muscles by tendons or fascia. The end of the muscle that moves during a contraction is the insertion, with the moving end being called the origin. Note that some muscles have more than one origin and insertion.

Integration (compound) The opposite of **isolation**. Movement that requires more than one joint and muscle to be involved, e.g. a squat.

Isolation The opposite of **integration**. A movement that requires only one joint and muscle to be involved, e.g. a bicep curl.

Interval training A type of training where you do blocks of high intensity exercise followed by a block of lower intensity (recovery) exercise. The blocks can be time based or marked by distance (in cardio training). Interval training is highly beneficial to both athletes and fitness enthusiasts as it allows them to subject their body to high-intensity activity in short, achievable bursts.

Intra-abdominal pressure (IAP) An internal force that assists in the stabilisation of the lumbar spine. This relates to the collective effects of pressure exerted on the structures of the diaphragm, transversus abdominis, multifidi and the pelvic floor.

Kettlebells In its original form a kettlebell was a cannonball with a handle on it. Modern versions are either know as 'classic' or 'pro grade' competition kettle-bells. The weight of kettlebells has traditionally been measured in 'poods' (a word derived from the Russian for 'Russian pound'), which equates to roughly 16kg to 1 pood. For beginners this is a challenging weight so, as kettlebells have become increasingly 'mass market', manufacturers have introduced lighter versions.

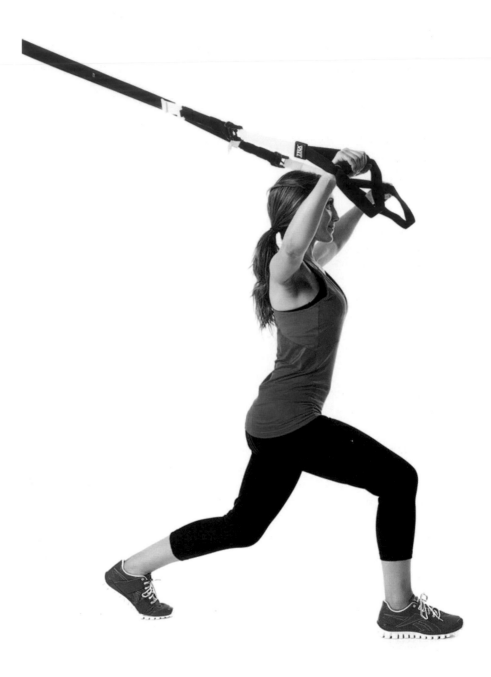

Most gyms will be equipped with cast iron or steel kettlebells ranging from 8kg to 332kg. If the kettlebells vary in size, they are 'classic' kettlebells, but if they are all the same size irrespective of what weight they are, then they are probably what is classed as being 'competition' or 'pro grade'. This means that no matter what weight you are lifting the dimensions of the weights are the same. This is important to people who enter lifting competitions because they can develop their technique using the standard shape and not have to re-learn or change their methods as they progress to heavier weights. The 'pro grade' kettlebells also have slimmer, smoother handles which help to minimise fatigue in your grip when performing high repetition sets.

Kinesiology The scientific study of the movement of our anatomical structure. It was only in the 1960s, with the creation of fixed weight machines, that we started to isolate individual muscles and work them one at a time. This is a step backwards in terms of kinesiology because in real life a single muscle rarely works in isolation.

Kinetic chain The series of reactions/forces throughout the nerves, bones, muscles, ligaments and tendons when the body moves or has a force applied against it.

Kyphosis Excessive curvature of the human spine. This can range from being a little bit round-shouldered to being in need of corrective surgery.

Lactic acid A by-product of muscle contractions. If lactic acid reaches a level higher than that which the body can quickly clear from the bloodstream, the person has reached their anaerobic threshold. Training at high intensity has the effect of delaying the point at which lactic acid levels cause fatigue.

Latissimus dorsi Two triangular-shaped muscles that run from the top of the neck and spine to the back of the upper arm and all the way into the lower back, also known as the lats.

Ligaments Connective tissues that attach bone to bone or cartilage to bone. They have fewer blood vessels passing through them than muscles, which makes them whiter (they look like gristle) and also slower to heal.

Lordosis Excessive curvature of the lower spine. Mild cases that are diagnosed early can often be resolved through core training and by working on flexibility with exercises best prescribed by a physiotherapist.

Massage Not just for pleasure or relaxation, this can speed up recovery and reduce discomfort after a hard training session. Massage can help maintain a range of motion in joints and reduce mild swelling caused by injury-related inflammation.

Magnesium An essential mineral that plays a role in over 300 processes in the body including in the cardiovascular system and tissue repair.

Maximum heart rate (MHR) The highest number of times the heart can contract (or beat) in one minute. A very approximate figure can be obtained for adults by using the following formula: 220 – current age = MHR. Athletes often exceed this guideline, but only because they have progressively pushed themselves and increased their strength over time.

Medicine ball Traditionally this was a leather ball packed with fibres to make it heavy. Modern versions are solid rubber, or filled with a heavy gel.

Mobility The ability of a joint to move freely through a range of motion. Mobility is very important because if you have restricted joint mobility and you start to load that area with weights, the chances are that you will compound the problem.

Muscular endurance (MSE) The combination of strength and endurance. The ability to perform many repetitions against a given resistance for a prolonged period. In strength training any more than 12 reps is considered MSE.

Negative-resistance training (NRT) Resistance training in which the muscles lengthen while still under tension. Lowering a barbell, bending down and running downhill are all examples. It is thought that this type of training increases muscle size more quickly than other types of training, but if you only ever do NRT you won't be training the body to develop usable functional strength.

Obliques The muscles on both sides of the abdomen that rotate and flex the torso. Working these will have no effect on 'love handles', which are areas of fat that sit above, but are not connected to, the obliques.

Origin All muscles are attached to bone or other muscles by tendons or fascia. The end of the muscle which is not moved during a contraction is the origin, with the moving end being called the insertion. Note that some muscles have more than one origin and insertion.

Overtraining Excessive amounts of exercise, intensity, or both, resulting in fatigue, illness, injury and/or impaired performance. Overtraining can occur in individual parts of the body or throughout, which is a good reason for keeping records of the training you do so you can see if patterns of injuries relate to a certain time or types of training you do throughout the year.

Patience With strength training – more than any other type of exercise – patience is essential. When you exercise the results are based on the ability of the body to 'change', which includes changes in the nervous system as well as progressive improvements in the soft tissues (muscles, ligaments and tendons). While it is not instantly obvious why patience is so important, it becomes clearer when you consider how, for example, the speed of change differs in the blood-rich muscles at a faster rate than the more avascular ligaments and tendons. Improvements take time, so be patient.

Pectorals The muscles of the chest, also known as the pecs. Working the pecs will have a positive effect on the appearance of the chest; however, despite claims, it is unlikely that working the pecs will have any effect on the size of female breasts, although it can make them feel firmer if the muscle tone beneath them is increased.

Pelvic floor (PF) Five layers of muscle and connective tissue at the base of the torso. The male and female anatomy differ in this area. However, strength and endurance are essential in the PF for both men and women if they are to attain maximum strength in the core. Most of the core training or stability products work the PF.

Periodisation Sums up the difference between a long-term strategy and short-term gains. Periodisation is where you plan to train the body for different outcomes over the course of a year or longer. The simplest version of this method would be where a track athlete worked on muscle strength and growth during the winter and then speed and maintenance of muscle endurance during the summer racing session.

Planes of motion The body moves through three planes of motion. Sagittal describes all the forward and backward movement; frontal describes the side to side movements; and transverse describes the rotational movements. In everyday life most of the movements we go through involve actions from all three planes all of the time –it is really only 'artificial' techniques, such as bicep curls and deltoid raises, that call upon just one plane at a time.

Plyometrics An explosive movement practised by athletes, for example, two-footed jumps over hurdles. This is not for beginners or those with poor levels of flexibility and/or a limited range of motion.

Prone Lying face down; also the standard description of exercises performed from a lying face down position. The opposite of supine (see below).

Protein A vital nutrient that needs to be consumed every day. Carbohydrates provide your body with energy, while protein helps your muscles to recover and repair more quickly after exercise. Foods high in protein include whey protein (which is a by-product of the dairy industry and is consumed as a shake), fish, chicken, eggs, dairy produce (such as milk, cheese and yoghurt), beef and soya.

Increased activity will increase your protein requirements. A lack of quality protein can result in loss of muscle tissue and tone, a weaker immune system, slower recovery and lack of energy. The protein supplements industry has developed many convenient methods for consuming protein in the form of powders, shakes and food bars, most of which contain the most easily digested and absorbable type of protein, whey protein.

Pyramid A programming method for experienced weight trainers. A set of the same exercises are performed at least three times, each set has progressively fewer repetitions in it, but greater resistance. When you reach the peak of the pyramid (heaviest weight) you then perform the same three sets again in reverse order. For example, going up the pyramid would ask for 15 reps with 10kg, 10 reps with 15kg, 5 reps with 20kg. Going down the pyramid would require 10 reps with 15kg, 15 reps with 10kg.

Quadriceps The groups of muscles at the front of the thighs, also known as the quads. They are usually the first four muscle names that personal trainers learn, but just in case you have forgotten, the four are: vastus intermedius, rectus femoris (that's the one that's also a hip flexor), vastus lateralis and vastus medialis.

Range of motion (ROM) The degree of movement that occurs at one of the body's joints. Without physio equipment it is difficult to measure a joint precisely, but you can easily compare the shoulder, spine, hip, knee and ankle on the left side with the range of motion of the same joints on the right side.

Reebok Core Board® A stability product that you predominately stand on. The platform has a central axis which creates a similar experience to using a wobble board; however, the Reebok Core Board® also rotates under tension so you can train against torsion and recoil.

Recoil The elastic characteristic of muscle when 'stretched' to return the body parts back to the start positions after a dynamic movement.

Recovery/rest The period when not exercising and the most important component of any exercise programme. It is only during rest periods that the body adapts to previous training loads and rebuilds itself to be stronger, thereby facilitating improvement. Rest is therefore vitally important for progression.

Repetitions How many of each movement you do, also known as reps. On training programmes you will have seen three numerical figures that you need to understand – **reps**, **sets** and **circuits**.

Repetition max (RM) The maximum load that a muscle or muscle group can lift. Establishing your RM can help you select the right amount of weight for different exercises and it is also a good way of monitoring progress.

Resistance training Any type of training with weights, including gym machines, barbells and dumbbells and bodyweight exercises.

Resting heart rate (RHR) The number of contractions (heartbeats) per minute when at rest. The average RHR for an adult is 72BPM, but for athletes it can be much lower.

Scapula retraction Not literally 'pulling your shoulders back', but that is a good cue to use to get this desired effect. Many people develop rounded shoulders, which when lifting weights puts them at a disadvantage because the scapular cannot move freely, so by lifting the ribs and squeezing the shoulder blades back the shoulder girdle is placed in a good lifting start position.

Sciatica Back pain which radiates through the spine, buttocks and hamstrings. Usually due to the sciatic nerve, which runs from the lower back and down the legs, being shortened due to pressure, rather than being a problem with the skeleton. Most often present in people who sit a lot. Core training, massage and flexibility exercises can frequently cure the problem.

Set A block of exercises usually put together to work an area of the body to the point of fatigue, so if you were working legs you may do squats, lunges and calf raises straight after each other, then repeat them again for a second 'set'.

Speed, agility and quickness (SAQ)® Although in fact a brand name, this has become the term used to describe a style of exercises or drills which are designed to improve speed, agility and quickness. Very athletic and dynamic, often including plyometric movements.

Stability ball (also gym ball, fitball and Swiss ball) The large balls extensively used for suitability training by therapists and in gyms. They are available in sizes 55–75cm. If you are using them for weight training always remember to add your weight and the dumbbell (or kettlebell) weight together to make sure the total weight doesn't exceed the safety limit of the ball.

Stretch A balanced approach to stretching is one of the most important elements of feeling good and reducing the likelihood of developing non-trauma soft tissue injuries. When we lift weight, the muscle fatigues and as a result at the end of the session the overall muscle (rather than individual fibres) can feel 'tight' or shortened. Doing a stretch will help return the muscle to its pre-exercise state. Dynamic stretching (rhythmic movements to promote optimum range of movement from muscle/joints) should be performed pre-workout. Static stretching performed after the session is productive as long as you dedicate enough time to each position, so give each section of the body worked at between 20 and 90 seconds of attention.

Suspension Spiral position (SS) The SS is a reference system that users of suspension systems can use to plot the appropriate position on the floor for their touch-points (hands or feet).

Superset Similar to a set, but each sequential exercise is performed with no rest in between. The moves in a superset are selected to ensure that they relate to each other, for example, an exercise that focused on shoulders and triceps, such as a shoulder press, would be followed by another shoulder/triceps move, such as dips.

Supine Lying face up, also the standard description of exercises performed from a lying face up position. The opposite of **prone**.

Tendon Connective tissue that attaches muscles to bones. Muscle and tendon tissue merge together progressively, rather than there being a clear line where tendon starts and muscle finishes. Like ligaments, a tendon has fewer blood vessels running through it and is less flexible than muscle tissue.

Time As a personal trainer, I have been asked many times, 'What is the best time of day to exercise?' The answer depends. If you are an athlete training almost every day perhaps twice a day, then I would say that strength training in the morning could be more productive than at other times due to the body clock and fluctuating hormone levels throughout the day. However, if the question is asked by a casual exerciser with an average diet and a job and busy lifestyle, my answer would be to exercise at any time of the day, as exercise is a productive use of your valuable free time.

Torsion Stress on the body when external forces twist it about the spinal axis.

Touch-points Where your body makes contact with a supporting structure (the floor, wall or suspension system). The smaller the touch-points, the more the balance demands increase for that exercise.

Training partner A training partner can be a person who keeps you company and motivates you while you exercise or they can also take the role of being your 'spotter' when you are lifting heavy weights. The role of a spotter is to hand and take the weights from you when you are fatigued from a heavy set of lifts. Choose your partner wisely; weights can be dangerous, so ensure they take the responsibility seriously.

Training shoes The best shoes to wear when lifting weights will have a combination of good grip and stability. Some athletes are now choosing to lift while wearing no or very thin-soled shoes on the basis that it will work the muscles in their feet more and therefore give greater results – if you do consider doing this, take a number of weeks to build up the amount you do barefoot to give the feet time to strengthen slowly. Athletes competing in powerlifting contests will wear performance shoes that give their feet increased support, however, these are not suitable for exercises in which the foot is moved.

Transversus abdominis A relatively thin sheet of muscle which wraps around the torso. This is the muscle that many people think they activate by following the instruction of 'pull your stomach in'; however, that movement is more likely to be facilitated by the main abdominals. For your information, a flat stomach is more likely to be achieved by simply standing up straight, as this ensures the correct distance between the ribs and pelvis.

Triceps Muscles at the back of the upper arms. They make up approximately two-thirds of the diameter of the upper arm, so if arm size is your goal, working the triceps will be a priority.

Vertebrae Individual bones that make up the spinal column. The intervertebral discs that sit between them are there to keep the vertebrae separated, cushion the spine and protect the spinal cord.

Vertical axis (VA) This is the shortest route from the anchor point to the ground beneath it. This line is used as a reference point to plot where an individual should place their hands or feet when suspended.

Vertical down force This is the pressure exerted on the handle or foot straps when they are loaded and also the force that has to be actively resisted between two or more touch-points. For example, when in a suspended press-up, the hands and feet are the touch-points and the vertical down force is apparent on the muscles of the core stabilisers.

Vertical Floor angle (V/F) A reference system to describe the angle of the user's body. For example, standing up straight is equal to a 90 degree V/F, then as you lean more towards the floor, your body and the floor create more acute angles. In this book, the most-used angles are 70, 45 and 30 degrees V/F.

VO_2 max The highest volume of oxygen a person can infuse into their blood during exercise. A variety of calculations or tests can be used to establish your VO_2 max; these include measuring the heart rate during and post aerobic activity. As each of these tests includes a measurement of the distance covered as well as the heart's reaction to activity, the most popular methods of testing VO_2 max are running, stepping, swimming or cycling for a set time and distance.

Warm-up The first part of any workout session that is intended to prepare the body for the exercise ahead of it. I find it is best to take the lead from the sports world and base the warm-up exactly on the movements you will do in the session. So if you are about to do weights rather than jog, go through some of the movements unloaded to prepare the body for the ranges of motion you will later be doing loaded.

Warm-down The slowing down or controlled recovery period after a workout session. A warm-down can include low-level cardio work to return the heart rate to a normal speed as well as stretching and relaxation.

Wobble board A circular wooden disc that you stand on with a hemisphere on one side. Originally used just by physiotherapists, they are now common in gyms and are used for stability training, core exercises and strengthening the ankle and/or rehabilitation from ankle injuries. Technology has been applied to this simple piece of equipment and there now exist progressive devices such as the Reebok Core Board® and the BOSU® (Both Sides Up), which achieve the same and more than the wooden versions.

X-training See **cross training**.

Yoga Probably the oldest form of fitness training in existence. Yoga has many different types (or styles) ranging from very passive stretching techniques through to explosive and dynamic style. It is often associated with hippy culture and 'yummy mummies', however, if you are doing any type of strength training, yoga will complement this nicely.

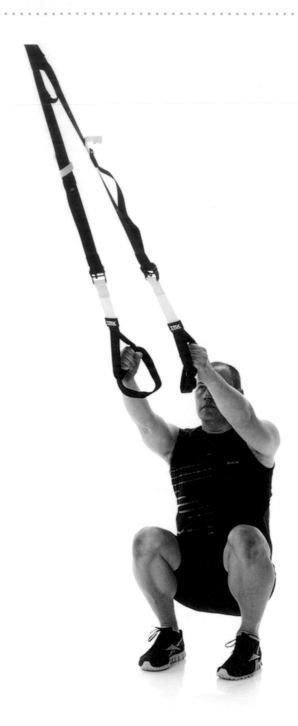

about the author

STEVE BARRETT is a former national competitor in athletics, rugby, mountain biking and sport aerobics. His career in the fitness industry as a personal trainer spans over 20 years. His work as a lecturer and presenter has taken him to 34 countries including the United States, Russia and Australia.

For many years Steve delivered Reebok International's fitness strategy and implementation via their training faculty Reebok University. He gained the title of Reebok Global Master Trainer, which is a certification that required a minimum of three years' studying, presenting and researching both practical and academic subjects. Between the years 2000 and 2008 in this role he lectured and presented to more than 20,000 fellow fitness professionals and students.

Steve played a key role in the development of the training systems and launch of two significant products in the fitness industry: the Reebok Deck and Reebok Core Board®. As a personal trainer, in addition to teaching the teachers and working with the rich and famous he has been involved in the training of many international athletes and sports personalities at Liverpool FC, Arsenal FC, Manchester United FC, the Welsh RFU, and UK athletics.

Within the fitness industry he has acted as a consultant to leading brand names, including Nestlé, Kelloggs, Reebok and Adidas.

His media experience includes being guest expert for the BBC and writing for numerous publications including *The Times*, the *Independent*, the *Daily Telegraph*, *Runner's World*, *Men's Fitness*, *Rugby News*, *Health & Fitness*, *Zest*, *Ultra-FIT*, *Men's Health UK* and *Australia* and many more.

Steve's expertise is in the development of logical, user-friendly, safe and effective training programmes. The work that he is most proud of, however, isn't his celebrity projects, but the changes to ordinary people's lives that never get reported.

Now that he has been teaching fitness throughout his 20s, 30s and 40s, he has developed a tremendous ability to relate to the challenges that people face to incorporate exercise into their lifestyle, and while the fitness industry expects personal trainers to work with clients for a short period of time, Steve has been working with many of his clients for nearly two decades, continuously evolving to meet their changing needs. His fun and direct approach has resulted in many couch potatoes running out of excuses and transforming into fitness converts.

www.Trade-secrets-of-a-Personal-Trainer.com

index